It's OK, MOM

The Nursing Home from a Sociological Perspective

It's OK, Mom

The Nursing Home
from a
Sociological Perspective

Joan Retsinas

Assistant Professor, Department of Family Medicine,
Brown University

The Tiresias Press, Inc.

Library of Congress Catalog Number: 86-050614
International Standard Book Number: 0-913292-14-1

Printed in U.S.A.

Contents

DEDICATION

To the people woven into my tapestry: Jennifer, Greg, and Amy, and to Nic, who helped weave the tapestry

Preface

The term "nursing home" seems an oxymoron, a contradiction in terms. On one hand, "nursing" evokes an image of uniformed credentialled staff, hospitals, admission and discharge requirements, and a hierarchy of medical personnel. The term also calls up the image of "patients," who, to use sociological jargon, fill the "sick role" so that they may become well. On the other hand, "home" evokes affection, a shared history, the daily routines of chores and conversation, and members, not patients. As a sociologist, I wanted to reconcile those two divergent images, to probe the extent to which a facility developed along a medical model could offer the requisites of a familial home.

The site of the research was The Nursing Home, a pseudonym for a 160-bed proprietary nursing home in New England. Data were collected in three separate statistical investigations. In the first, data were gathered from staff interviews and patient charts to probe the frequency of visitors, the emotional feelings of staff toward residents, and staff knowledge of resident pasts. That research was conducted in the summer of 1982 and focused on 130 residents who had lived at the home at least 5 months and 54 staff members who had worked at the home at least 4 months. (In this book, this sample of residents and staff is referred to as Sample A.) The second investigation focused on friendships among residents. The research used staff interviews to delineate friendship patterns of 145 residents living in The Nursing Home during the summer of 1984 (Sample B). Although The Nursing Home houses 160 residents, the research omitted the very new residents. Finally, to disentangle the factors important in patient discharges, data were gathered from the case histories of the 415 residents (Sample C) discharged from 1978 through June 1984.

The background to this research has been a steady drumbeat of scandal. Newspapers and legislative commissions have portrayed a sizeable proportion of nursing homes as dirty, negligent, and generally abysmal. According to a recent Senate investigation, one-third of nursing homes fail to meet Federal health, care, and safety standards, and about a thousand of these are in gross violation of those standards.*

The Nursing Home is among the two-thirds of the adequate nursing homes. Once every two months an inspector from the state health department visits it unannounced, and The Nursing Home addresses the occasional complaints (for instance, missing dentures or a soiled gerichair). Until 1986, moreover, the inspector from the state health department annually visited every Medicaid patient in all nursing homes throughout the state. (Starting with 1986, the state inspector is required to visit only a sampling of Medicaid patients.) The inspector was supposed to talk individually with each Medicaid patient. If the patient was comatose, the inspector ver-

---

*Editorial, *The New York Times,* S4:24, June 15, 1986.

ified first-hand the patient's condition, in addition to reviewing the patient's chart. Rarely has the state found deficits in The Nursing Home.

The Nursing Home, however, is not a model of excellence. Its architectural layout is unimaginative. Its social schedule offers no extraordinary activities. Its staff consists largely of aides, many of whom doubtless have no notion of "gerontological rehabilitation" or "induced dependence." Writers looking for an extraordinary home will bypass The Nursing Home. This ordinary nursing home, however, has competent, caring staff. I am grateful to them for graciously finding time in hectic schedules to answer questions and complete charts as I put their facility under the harsh scrutiny of statistical analysis. Indeed, staff warmth, enthusiasm, and caring marked such a contrast with both the popular and professional nursing home literature that, as a sociologist, I wanted to investigate the seeming paradox of a "nursing home."

Some of the data on staff knowledge of, and affect toward, residents (Chapters 4 and 5) appeared in *The California Sociologist*, v. 6:129-150, 1983. The tables that outline friendship patterns in the nursing home (Chapter 3) appeared in *The Gerontologist* 25: 376-381, 1985. Some data on the discharge track of residents (Chapter 7) appear in *The Gerontologist* 26:431–436, 1986, and some will appear in the *International Journal of Aging and Human Development* in 1987. These data are used with permission. The quotation at the beginning of Chapter 3 is from "Choruses from 'The Rock' " in *Collected Poems 1909-1962 by T.S. Eliot*, copyright 1935 by Harcourt Brace Jovanovich, copyright © 1963, 1964 by T.S. Eliot. Reprinted by permission of the publisher.

— J.R.

Chapter 1

"*Through a Glass, Darkly...*"

If the title of this book, "It's OK, Mom," seems unduly optimistic to those who have anguished over sending their relative to live in a nursing home, it is because nursing homes are not necessarily as bleak as we imagine them to be. And we imagine them as bleak. If you gave a random assortment of people—even a random assortment of sociologists—a word-association test on "nursing home," the likely responses would be "abandonment," "dismal," "senile," "warehouse," "graft," "abuse," "institution." If you then asked these same people whether they wanted to end their lives in a nursing home, they emphatically would say no. The popular image of a nursing home is of a geriatric black hole where people, isolated from friends and families, await death.

When we look at nursing homes, however, what we see is refracted by the lenses of our experience, our perceptions of normality, the values of our time, and the visions of contemporaries. Grounded in our own time and place, we see nursing homes from a distinct perspective—one that colors our images, no matter how conscientiously we profess an analytical, value-free, non-judgmental stance.

Artists exemplify how the refraction of vision reflects both contemporary values and individual creativity. By technique, choice of subjects, and scale, artists evoke their epoch—the careful domesticity of 18th century Dutch art, the opulent baroque figures, the cubism of Postimpressionism; yet even within the same epoch, different artists, interpreting the same scene, offer distinctive versions. What we see reflects, to a large measure, the lenses through which we gaze.

Similarly, the interpretation of "reality" by historians and anthropologists reflects their own values and biases. Tracing the American Revolution, a feminist historian[1] uses different terms and suggests different motivations than would a more traditional historian. Richard III's persistent reputation as the murderer of his young nephews reflects not necessarily the "truth" of the tale, but the biases of recording historians.[2] Commentators' analyses of contemporary events, such as the famine in Ethiopia or the future for nuclear energy, reflect their own ideological stance.

Even science, that supposedly value-free pursuit of pure truth, reflects the visions and values of its practitioners. In *The Structure of Scientific Revolutions,* Thomas Kuhn[3] introduced the notion of a paradigm. For Kuhn, a paradigm represents a particular perspective on reality. If reality is construed as a kaleidoscope of people, events, and empirical facts, then a paradigm represents one setting of the kaleidoscope. If reality is a puzzle, the paradigm determines which pieces of the puzzle are to be grouped, analyzed, and regrouped. At any point in time, scientists share one world-view and work from one paradigm, testing hypotheses and analyzing data that complement that view. This is called "Normal Science," with most scientists working on similar parts of the puzzle, asking similar questions, and testing each others' conclusions. During such a period scientists seem to be "building upon the shoulders of giants" as persistent research augments knowledge. Kuhn challenged the implicit progressivism of "Normal Science," however, by stressing that any paradigm contains questions that research within that paradigm cannot answer. When these unanswered questions, or "anomalies," accumulate to a critical point, the dominant paradigm will fall, to be replaced by a new paradigm, one capable of explaining the anomalies and, generally, one espoused by younger scientists not so thoroughly indoctrinated in the old paradigm. In what Kuhn dubbed "paradigmatic revolutions," Copernican astronomy supplanted the astronomy of Ptolemy, and Einsteinian physics supplanted Newtonian physics. A paradigm is not "wrong," but simply inadequate to explain certain questions. As historians of science have noted, moreover, scientists have an intellectually and economically vested interest in their paradigm. In *The Double Helix*, Watson[4] laid bare the political maneuvering behind "scientific" research essential to the understanding of DNA. Often scientists "see" what they are trained to see, what they expect to see, what their colleagues have seen, or what they want to see.

Not surprisingly, then, our visions of the nursing home are no less skewed by the lenses through which we gaze—lenses clouded by the "dominant" paradigm of institutionalism, by an artificial continuum of nursing home/family, and by our own attitude toward aging and death. We cannot readily discard the lenses through which we view reality; indeed, Kuhn's notion of paradigmatic revolutions emphasizes the fact that reality is so multi-faceted, so kaleidoscopic, that one must work within paradigms to construct meaningful explanations for the world we inhabit. "Non-paradigmatic" science or "value-free" historical interpretation are not possible. We can, however, recognize the paradigms under which we work, the values that guide our research, the attitudes that shape our interpretations of reality. To understand the nursing home, we must first examine the lenses through which we gaze.

The Institutional Paradigm

To use Kuhn's notion of paradigms, most research on nursing homes has reflected an "institutional" paradigm. In *Asylums*, Erving Goffman[5] set forth in bleak clarity the outline of an archetypal "total institution," and this vision of a total institution has guided both research and researchers, who have looked at nursing homes as examples of institutions, at nursing home residence as a kind of institutionalization, and at the impact of residence as inherently debilitating.

In an archetypal institution like Goffman's asylum, dehumanization begins upon admission, when the individual is stripped of clothing, watch, jewelry, wallet, money, and any other material links to the world "outside." Since the individual is to become an inmate, his outer garb must reflect his new identity. The metaphorical stripping away of past identity will continue throughout the inmate's stay. In describing the formation of self-image, G. Herbert Mead[6] maintained that we see ourselves through the eyes of others. Those images, reflected back as in a "looking glass," underlay our own images of ourselves. In a variation of Mead's looking glass, the inmate will live among staff and fellow inmates who will recognize him only as "the case in 103;" his prior social roles, as worker, spouse, parent, friend, are no longer salient. Within the world of the institution he must construct a new social identity, based upon the role of inmate. The successful inmate may learn to use the meager resources of the institution (cigarettes, for instance) to gain status because his former status will no longer be recognized. Physically isolated from relatives and friends, the inmate receives visits at specified times in specified places, so that relationships active "before" the inmate entered the institution become formalized into visitor and visitee.

In a total institution the inmate forfeits responsibility for decisions about his life. The administrator will determine the what, where, when, how, and with whom for the inmate. Routines are prescribed: the "good" inmate complies with a prescribed *modus operandi*; the "bad" inmate asserts independence. Meals, times of bathing, recreational activities, room locations—all are for the most part set. The inmate may have limited autonomy to choose chicken or fish for lunch, but rarely the timing of meals or the option to eat outside the institution. And individuals allowed to ignore institutional timetables often must suffer consequences. The inmate who is permitted to sleep late, for instance, may forego breakfast.

If the institution transforms the individual into an inmate, it similarly dehumanizes staff, who become formal adjuncts to the larger bureaucratic entity. Largely untrained, staff have specific tasks to accomplish—usually custodial tasks. Routinized order dominates a total institution, and staff are instrumental in the realization of that order. Consequently, staff-inmate relationships lack empathy. Indeed, affection and love do not belong within the world of the institution. Staff function as combination police-custodians, and while inmates may grow fond of one another, cavalier reshuffling of inmate rooms and routines is not designed to foster intimacy. If affection between inmates impedes efficient running of the institution, moreover, then affection would be discouraged.

Goffman presented an "ideal type" of total institution. Individual asylums vary in the extent to which residents retain ties with the outside world, with the autonomy allowed inmates, with the attitudes of staff, and with the completeness of the "mantle" of inmate. The model Goffman drew, however, clearly set forth the requisites of an institution; and researchers, looking at nursing homes from such an institutional paradigm, have analyzed the resident's isolation from family and friends, the passive role of resident-patient, the formalized staff-resident relationships, the limited autonomy allowed residents, and the lack of affection between caregivers and those receiving care. Measuring nursing homes against Goffman's model, researchers have pronounced them debilitating, sterile, and dehumanizing[7]—a portrait that stresses the deficits of nursing home residence. Not surprisingly, policy makers sensitive to this research have stressed the need to keep people out of institutions, not simply because it is cheaper to keep people in the community, but because it is "better" for the individuals themselves.

Newspaper exposes have substantiated the image of the nursing home as an institution where people deteriorate. Journalists have focused on the filth, the lack of medical safeguards, the carelessness of staff, the abuse by greedy owners, and the fraudulent bilking of Medicaid, Medicare, and patient families. Listening to Congressional testimony, we conjure up avaricious physicians who submit fraudulent bills, owners eager only for a tax write-off, abusive and/or larcenous and/or poorly-trained and/or overworked and/or aloof staff, crowded facilities in violation of building and fire safety codes, unpalatable food, and apathetic, inert residents waiting only to die.[8]

An institution offers few possibilities of escape. In *One Flew Over the Cuckoo's Nest*,[9] audiences cheered when Jack Nicholson challenged the misanthropic Nurse Ratchet, threw the well-ordered asylum into chaos, and tried to escape, thereby affirming our hope that individuals can prevail over the Kafkaesque horror that is the institution. Nursing homes have few patients likely to revolt, and we make no heroic movies about nursing home residents. Indeed, one of the few movies to focus on senescence, *Going in Style*,[10] featured three elderly bank robbers who believed that wealth would insure them an exciting old age. After two of the men died, the surviving robber gave the bounty to his friend's son. From prison, the elderly man gently assured the son that jail offered food, shelter, safety—the same amenities, in fact, that he would find in a nursing home.

"Be It Ever So Humble"

If we see the nursing home as a horrid institution, with the derogatory connotations that word carries, we see "the family" through far kinder lenses. If people gathered around a dining room table were asked to free associate with the word "family," they would likely mention "affection," "support," "loyalty," "obligations," "responsibilities," and "households." The "family" evokes generally positive connotations although actual families may grotesquely distort the ideal. We hear often of child abuse, elderly abuse, marital violence, incest, child abandonment, rivalries—all testifying to a reality that mocks Norman Rockwell notions of togetherness. Nevertheless, we see the family, at least the "healthy, functioning" family, as "good" for the individual. Impoverished unmarried mothers need employed husbands; boys need a male role model; girls need a female model; children need parental involvement; and, finally, the elderly person needs loving, devoted children.

Since changing demographic patterns have only recently made the four-generation family common, we have limited historical experience with it; nevertheless, we persist in believing that the Norman Rockwell multigenerational portrait represents, perhaps not the family as it is, but certainly the family as it should be, as we want it to be, as it could be if we were only more dedicated, more loving, more unselfish.[11] The field of housing exemplifies the schism between reality and our notion of the ideal. On one hand, architects and planners like multi-generational communities. One architect writes: "They (the elderly) need adventure and excitement, something to look forward to, something to make tomorrow different from today, and a sense that they are part of it. These things are not as apt to occur in an old folks home, even though it is small and called by a different name. Anticipation and involvement with all ages helps keep people young."[12] On the other hand, elderly-housing complexes report waiting lists. The popularity of both federally-subsidized projects and costlier retirement communities nestled in geriatric havens far from children and grandchildren suggests that at least some elderly people are declining to pose for the Norman Rockwell portrait. Surveys, moreover, show that today most elderly people do not want to depend upon their children.[13] As for today's children, when I asked my class of college undergraduates whether they wanted their parents to live with them, they paled.

The lines of "family," moreover, have blurred in the last decade. Divorce, remarriage, stepchildren, half-children—relationships are, both legally and emotionally, less emphatically delineated. In TV's Waltons we can easily identify the elders, their children, their grandchildren; but in contemporary families the ties that bind may no longer bind so tightly. When an 80-year-old man is incapacitated from a stroke, is his wife of ten years the primary caregiver? If she herself is frail, do her children assume the responsibility for their stepfather, even though they may barely know him? Are the children from his first marriage responsible for him? If he was divorced and estranged from their mother when they were growing up, must those children, now adults, still act as caregivers, regardless of the dearth of affection? As individual geneological diagrams have grown more complicated, so too the demarcation of families has grown more difficult.

Nevertheless, in contrast to the bleak institution, we have exalted the supportive family. Indeed, we have constructed a continuum, with the institution at one end and the family at the other. In this view, the institution has caregivers intent on performing instrumental tasks for pay; the family has children caring for beloved parents. In an institution, the individual becomes a "case"; in the family, the individual remains a parent, grandparent, and friend. Institutional life allows little personal autonomy; at home the individual is responsible for setting his own schedule. Residents of an institution are isolated from the community; members of a household are involved in the community. Institutional food is appalling; home-cooked food, nourishing. Within an institution people sit apathetically waiting for visitors; at home people socialize with each other. Even the nursing home scandals of fraud, avarice, and abuse that investigators have unearthed shock, but do not truly surprise, readers. Within a facility where people have no emotional bonds—indeed, where financial obligations usually underlie caregiving, the abuses seem an unfortunate offshoot, if not the norm. To guard against abuses within nursing homes, we rely on governmental oversight, not upon unstated moral codes. Reports of a kind, loving nursing home where staff bonded with their charges and where residents enjoyed living with each other would seem aberrant. On the other hand, families are expected to be loving and caring. When journalists unearth instances of family abuse, we shudder and are surprised. To regulate family relationships we rely largely on unstated codes of conduct, not on governmental edicts. In a kind of dualistic, Manichaean image, we have made "the family" into the antithesis of "the institution."

This Manichaean dichotomy haunts families who "put" relatives into nursing homes. Even the word "put" suggests a spurning, a casting forth, as the family that is insufficiently familial resorts to the nursing home for the relative whom they cannot/will not care for themselves. The reality, of course, is that many elderly people consciously participate in the decision to enter a nursing home,[14] that many families have exhausted all their financial and emotional resources in caregiving,[15] and that a severely demented person can destroy the most Walton-like family. Nevertheless, families struggle with guilt as they talk to administrators, sign the required forms, and move their parents' possessions from the "community" home, the "real" home, to this new, institutional one. Nursing home social workers try constantly to assuage familial guilt. Progressive nursing homes offer family support groups, partly to acclimate relatives to the home, mostly to help them share their feelings with other guilt-ridden people.

Guilt not only makes families heartbroken when they admit a parent to a nursing home. It also skews their perspective on nursing home life when they visit. Journal articles discuss uncaring, aloof, misanthropic staff; but nursing home staff themselves, on their coffee breaks, discuss omnipresent occupational hazards: the families whose overzealous visits hinder the new resident,[16] or the relative who translates guilt into hysterical fault-finding. The relative who is convinced that he has abandoned his parent looks to negate his guilt by finding neglect and/or abuse. Very critical families may choose to transfer their relatives. Physicians claim that the never-to-be-satisifed patient who travels from physician to physician suffers from Munchausen syndrome. In a variation of Munchausen syndrome, some residents are transferred from nursing home to nursing home until their families find the nursing home that best resolves their guilt.

Some of us may have watched relatives enter nursing homes. Some may foresee a "nursing home decision" for elderly relatives. Still others may have known families who evaluate the home through their own anguish. An institutional paradigm is the intellectual lens through which we see nursing homes. Scholars, gerontologists, researchers, and investigators have told us the countless ways in which nursing home residence represents in-stitutionalization, with all its negative connotations. The family-institution continuum, where the family repre-sents the optimum home for the elderly "in the best of all worlds," is an emotional lens through which we gaze at nursing homes. We see the home as our friends and relatives have seen it, as we ourselves imagine we will see it when we sign a relative into an institution.

Discharge

We also see in the nursing home a foreboding of death—not an irrational foreboding since most long-term residents will die there. Many residents are ill; indeed, the implementation of Diagnostic Related Groupings (DRGs) for hospital Medicare reimbursement has increased nursing homes' census of the moribund as hospitals seek to discharge patients quickly. In the cheeriest nursing home, with the most ebullient staff, we recognize that nursing home residence marks a prelude to death for most patients. Optimistically, state regulations force nursing home social workers to prepare regular "discharge plans" for residents. A discharge plan specifies whether the resident will return to the community, whether such a return depends upon specific conditions, or whether the placement is permanent. "Shortstayers"—often, people admitted for therapy after a hip replacement or people admitted only while a caregiver is absent—generally enter with "positive" discharge plans and return to the community. "Permanent placements," in contrast, usually leave only to go to the hospital and die. People who die in the nursing home are, euphemistically, labelled "discharged"; but they are discharged to a mortuary.

The fact that residents will die is not startling. Shakespeare called death "a necessary end" that "will come when it will come." In the nursing home corridors, however, we glimpse the pain, the deterioration, the diminished faculties that may precede death; and this graphic, sensual reminder startles Americans, who value youth and activity and independence. We like to think that senescence need not be painful, disfiguring, or unpleasant, and, indeed, would prefer to die while fully competent and active. Ancient Dinka spearmasters[17] could choose the time, place, and manner of their death. Like them, we too would like to choose our own *ars moriendi* or, if not, we would at least like to remain lucid and in control.[18] The reality that some people will not die quickly, suddenly, and painlessly troubles us. In the media elderly people are usually attractive, alert, mobile, able to feed and dress themselves. If they die on television or in the movies, death takes no longer than the timing of the show.

Many people are not so fortunate as movie or TV characters. They deteriorate, suffer, and grow dependent on the ministrations of others. Even famous historical figures who lived into their eighties did not necessarily escape pain or disability. Benjamin Franklin, who took opium to alleviate gout, wrote George Washington, "For my own personal ease I should have died years ago, but though those years have been spent in excruciating pain, I am pleased that I have lived them . . ."[19] Gilbert Stuart depicted the costumes, the wigs, the graceful stances, but not the feebleness or the pain of elderly Colonial heroes. Obviously, some people age gracefully, remaining healthy, functioning, and attractive. Georgia O'Keefe, Pablo Picasso, Marc Chagall—all were octogenarians. Soviet leaders have traditionally been in their seventies. Oliver Wendell Holmes studied Greek when he was eighty. The examples of graceful longevity, however, do not negate the existence of people who age far less gracefully. These people—the ungraceful aged[20]—live in nursing homes.

For these residents, death is inexorable. Neither medical magic nor vitamins nor positive thinking will restore flexibility to muscles, vitality to gait, or lucidity to consciousness. We cannot help most residents improve, but we can care humanely for them, hoping to make their end as painless, as joyful, and as peaceful as possible. To some extent, when we gaze down nursing home corridors, we glimpse our own mortality—a glimpse that in turn colors our perception of the nursing home. When we grieve for the person bedridden with cancer, we also grieve for ourselves. Filled with ill people about to die, the nursing home seems a harbinger of our own possible fate. Gerard Manley Hopkins[21] cautioned a young girl who was watching autumn leaves fall:

> *Margaret, are you grieving*
> *Over Goldengrove unleaving?*
> . . . .
> *It is the blight man was born for,*
> *It is Margaret you mourn for.*

Our own troubled anguish at this harbinger of our end reflects our deepest feelings about death. When we look at the nursing home, we confront at the same time our own mortality. The lenses through which we gaze reflect this recognition, just as they reflect our expectations of familial responsibilities and our notion that the nursing home represents an "institution," with all the connotations that word carries.

A Family Paradigm

This book seeks to show a very ordinary nursing home, but to show it through lenses that reflect, not an institutional paradigm, but a family paradigm. Instead of probing the extent to which the nursing home meets the criteria of a total institution, the research probes the extent to which the nursing home meets the criteria of a family.

At first, the notion of the nursing home as a familial community may seem far-fetched. A hospital-modelled facility that provides nursing care, usually for profit, seems by definition incapable of providing the camaraderie, the love, and the caring we expect within a home. Thus "nursing home" appears as contradictory a term as "Unloving Care,"[22] or "Tender Loving Greed,"[23] the titles of two derogatory exposes of nursing homes. To think of the nursing home as a possible home, we must discard the family-institution continuum.

The first step in discarding the continuum is to recognize, not how the nursing home fits the model of an archetypal institution, but how the nursing home deviates from that model. Unlike a total institution, the nursing home does not deliberately try to isolate the individual from family and friends. On the contrary, family visits and involvement are encouraged. Some residents—"expanders"—may even have more contact with other people after they enter the nursing home than before.[24] Residents able to leave for a day or a weekend may do so. Many residents enter only for a short period of time, then return to the community. Residents frequently transfer to other homes. No regulations bar residents from bringing family pictures or other mementos with them. Nursing home residents wear their own clothes, not hospital clothes. Often residents choose nursing homes where they already know other residents. Individual nursing homes vary in the "totality" of their institutional environment. Although the nursing home fits some criteria of Goffman's asylum, the fit is imperfect, and researchers might justifiably step back from the "institutional" paradigm that has dominated research and analyze the extent to which the nursing home functions as a family.

Family systems analysts[25] have outlined characteristics of an archetypal family. A family is bounded from the outside world. Boundaries may be rigid, chaotic, or flexible, but typically some differentiation exists to give individuals a family identity, so that even while individuals participate in the larger community, they remain involved with the family. Family members care about each other. Although in some families the "affective involvement" and "affective responsiveness" may be insufficient or excessive, the norm for family relationships prescribes emotional bonding, not the instrumental objectivity that is supposed to dominate relationships in an institution. Similarly, although cohesion between members may range from emmeshed to disengaged, cohesion remains a characteristic of families, as does adaptability, which can range from rigid to chaotic. Family members know each others' pasts; nobody remains, at least within the familial context, a "stranger." Actual families have their own division of labor, their own leadership structure, their own philosophical values. Although the family of procreation and the family of origin are the most recognized units, the functions of a family need not be limited to nuclear families.

As Kuhn noted, the choice of a paradigm determines the questions that researchers ask. Working with an institutional paradigm, researchers have analyzed the adverse effects of institutionalization upon residents. From a family paradigm, a researcher can ask different questions, analyze different data, test different hypotheses.

The research reported in this book is set within a family paradigm. It analyzes the extent to which residents retain the identities they had before they entered the nursing home, the ties they have with the outside community, the bonds that exist between staff and residents, the friendships that develop among residents, the feelings residents have about their new home, and the changes in residents' functioning while they live in the nursing home. In a sense, the research represents a search for a familial community within the facility known as a "nursing home." Researchers searching for an institution have found that the nursing home is indeed one. Here, the research seeks to find, amidst the white-coated aides and vinyl corridors of a very ordinary facility, a kind of home. The research is sociological; hence, the tools include both open-ended and structured interviews with staff, case records of patients, discharge rates, and transfer patterns. By analyzing the statistical evidence from many staff members and many patients, the research discovers that different lenses will yield a meaningful picture of nursing home life.

Chapter 2

An Ordinary Nursing Home

The search for a familial community begins inauspiciously in an ordinary nursing home. The Nursing Home (a pseudonym) is a proprietary 160-bed nursing home in New England that offers all levels of care, from self-care to Skilled Nursing. The home accepts Medicaid as well as private-paying patients; indeed, over three-quarters of its residents generally receive Medicaid subsidies. The Nursing Home is neither a model geriatric rehabilitation center nor a flagrantly profitable warehouse for the dying. It looks, feels, even smells like a host of other nursing homes.

It does not, however, feel like a home. It is an amalgam. From investors' perspective, it is a financial corporate entity. From state regulators' perspective, it is a medical facility. From staff perspective, it is a labor-intensive workplace. Only for residents does it purport to be a home.

The Blueprint: Neither Bricks nor Mortar . . .

Physically the structure, built in the late 1970's, resembles a two-story 1950's motel designed by hospital administrators. With four units on two long horizontal wings,

27

the building is neither charming nor functional. Cramped in the middle of each unit is a nursing station, where staff use a table for paper-work, coffee breaks, and conferences. Patient rooms line the long corridors. Each floor has one dining room, which doubles regularly as a chapel, occasionally as an auditorium. Between floors are stairways, not ramps. Two elevators serve all units. On the first floor are the offices of the administrator, the receptionist, the comptroller, and the social worker. A small conference room is on the first floor. Nursing offices are on the second floor.

Patient rooms are sparse and hospital-like. Although the home has eight single rooms, most rooms have two beds and one window. Typical of such rooms, one resident will always be able to see outside if s/he wants; the other resident will be trapped on the darker side while in the room since, as in a hospital, a sliding curtain separates the beds. Each resident has one nursing station call button, one night table, one small chair, one large chair, one closet, and three drawers of the single bureau. Residents share a sink and mirror. Each private room has its own bathroom; two double rooms (four residents) share one bathroom. Each floor, however, has two extra bathrooms for patients. The home uses drapes, not blinds on windows, so that light cannot filter in when they are closed. The rooms are just large enough to accommodate the bureau, chairs, night tables, sink, and beds.

Administrators encourage residents to bring memorabilia from home; yet the paucity of wall and counter space effectively limits residents from making the rooms reflect their families, lives, or interests. Every resident has an afghan for the bed. If neither the patient's family nor the patient can supply one, The Nursing Home's social worker will find one. Residents may and do bring comfortable chairs from home to replace the in-

stitution's chairs; indeed, resident families are urged to
bring either a recliner or a rocking chair; yet, again, the
cramped quarters leave little space for such furniture.

At the front entrance to The Nursing Home a
wooden bench faces the street, and residents able to get
there may sit outside. For residents in walkers or wheelchairs, access depends upon finding a staff member
willing to take them outside. For ambulatory residents,
access generally requires some minimal assistance, if not
from staff, then from visitors. Although the entrance to
the home has no stairs, the entrance has heavy doors,
which a frail resident cannot easily open. The Nursing
Home has recently added an outside sitting area at a
rear corner of the home. The area contains perhaps 20
lawn chairs grouped around a square of concrete. Again,
residents able to get there may sit outside, but the area
is immediately accessible to residents on only one unit;
and even residents on that unit will generally need staff
assistance to open doors. The second floor has no porch
or solarium. The most incapacitated patients live on the
second floor, where they have no access to the outdoors.
Second-floor residents do get outside, but only if staff
and/or family members take them.

The home provides a few communal living spaces.
One large living room, with comfortable chairs and an
attractive carpet, flanks the entrance. The second floor
has a smaller living room. Both living rooms have television sets and the downstairs living room has a piano. In
the downstairs living room visitors and staff contribute
discarded magazines. These rooms are rarely used; and
since they are not immediately accessible to unit staff in
the nursing stations, staff cannot readily see residents
who are in the communal living rooms. Consequently,
staff are reluctant to let patients who might wander or
patients who might need help quickly or patients who

are incontinent—in short, a great many patients—sit in
the living rooms. The second floor has a small chapel,
seating 20. At the end of the first floor, in an annex, is
a pool table, rarely used. People strolling through this
nursing home would see residents either in their rooms
or lined up against the walls of the corridors. In the
main living room they might see an occasional visitor or
a prospective resident's family waiting to meet the social
worker.

The floors are white vinyl, with black stripes along
the borders. The almond-colored walls display paintings
of rural scenes and still lifes, although for the first two
years of The Nursing Home's existence the walls were
bare. The walls of the patients' rooms do not have paintings or posters supplied by The Nursing Home, but residents may hang their own pictures.

The kitchen is on the first floor. Kitchen staff will
bring meals to residents and clear away trays, but the
residents themselves have no direct access to kitchen
facilities. Each unit, however, has a small refrigerator, a
hot plate, and a toaster, so that unit staff may offer an
occasional snack to residents. Residents on the self-care
unit may get their own juice and crackers; residents may
not use the hot plates and toasters.

Even though the social work intake case histories
for many residents cite gardening as an avocation, the
home is remarkably bare of greenery. Patients' families
may bring plants or flowers to individual rooms, but The
Nursing Home itself offers neither greenery nor colorful
floral arrangements, except for a few plants in the living
rooms. The front yard consists of a circular driveway
bordered by a patch of grass and scattered shrubs; the
back yard, of a large asphalt parking lot bordered by a
larger patch of grass and a few evergreen bushes. At one
corner of the back yard, near the parking lot, is the small

rear patio area. The grounds do have both spring and summer flowers.

The Nursing Home Day

The day begins at 7:00 a.m., when day staff begin their shift. Although in some nursing homes the night staff rouse residents, at The Nursing Home residents may sleep until 7:00, when staff ready them for the day, which consists largely of prayer, bingo, meals, and television, interrupted by regularly weekly sessions with the hairdresser—a schedule that one gerontologist[1] dubbed the standard nursing home regimen.

Religious services dominate the social schedule. Each Sunday a priest and a Protestant minister conduct separate services in the ground floor dining room. The Nursing Home's small chapel is used mainly for individual meditation or family talks. In addition, since 65% of the residents are Catholic, on Tuesdays volunteers from the neighborhood parish lead the rosary in the first-floor dining room, where a 10-inch plaster figurine of Mary is lifted onto a dining room table. Also on Tuesdays, a Baptist minister conducts services. Since many residents participated actively in their community churches, clergy regularly visit former parishioners. Although some residents could leave the nursing home for religious services in their own churches, no church expressly includes these residents within its congregation, either by using volunteer drivers or by scheduling a van for Sunday mornings.

Religious services reflect various religious holidays, but not patient deaths. Although some nursing homes schedule memorial services for residents who have died, this nursing home does not.

Bingo is a staple of the recreational agenda. Three times a week a resident becomes the caller for nursing home bingo games, which are held at different times in both dining rooms. An average of 25 residents will attend. The usual prize is a quarter.

Meals are the major social events. Patients fed intravenously or by G-tubes do not eat in the dining room, and Intermediate Care Facility (ICF I) residents may eat in their rooms if they choose. Self-care (ICF II) residents, however, must eat in one of the two dining rooms. Indeed, the dining rooms are the hubs of the nursing home. Between religious services, bingo games, and meals, staff continually usher people into and out of the dining rooms. During meals residents have the opportunity to make friends, to talk, to see other residents, and to learn nursing home gossip. Staff will help feed residents who need assistance. Although the serving of a meal may take only 30 minutes, "mealtime" itself may last up to 90 minutes. Since staff must wheel and help residents to the dining room, they may begin marshalling people as early as 11:30 for a 12:00 lunch. At this nursing home meals are served at 8 a.m., noon, and 5 p.m.—a schedule influenced by federal regulations[2] which require a set number of hours to elapse between meals, so that nursing homes anxious to economize on staff time do not schedule meals close together. In many nursing homes breakfast begins early, so that the night shift is responsible for rousing residents.

In nursing homes generally, institutional food is a perpetual cause for lament, both by visitors and residents. In fact, research[3] on the agenda items of nursing home resident councils suggests that residents are primarily concerned, not with the management of the nursing home, the schedule of social activities, or the institutional rules, but simply with the variety and quality of food. Since the days revolve around mealtimes and since food provides one of the few sensory pleasures, resident concern is justifiable.

The menu at this nursing home is bland, yet nutritious. The main luncheon courses for one week consisted of ham, braised beef cubes on rice, breaded veal cutlet, turkey divan, fried steak, filet of sole, and chicken croquettes. The Nursing Home serves the main meal in the middle of the day because staff feel that residents who go to bed early sleep better after a light, rather than a heavy, meal. Supper varies, from hot dogs to bologna and cheese sandwiches to a cheese omelette (see sample menu). Fresh fruit and uncooked vegetables are rare, but then many residents prefer not to eat salads. As required by federal regulations, the home offers evening snacks. For birthdays, holidays, or special occasions the kitchen staff will produce punch and a cake. In the summer evenings the dietary staff will occasionally offer lemonade to residents and visiting relatives. For special holidays, guests may arrange in advance to eat with their relatives; for regular meals visitors generally do not eat in the dining hall or patient rooms, although occasionally a visitor will stay. For holiday meals guests must pay, while the occasional mealtime guest at a regular meal is generally served without prior arrangements and at no charge.

The second most popular destination is the beauty parlor. If the dining room is the focal mecca of the nursing home, the beauty parlor ranks second. Nursing homes generally contract with a hairdresser on a consignment basis. Since every resident, even those on Medicaid, has some monthly discretionary spending money, every female resident is a potential customer. Indeed, one writer[4] noted the not-uncommon phenomenon of an unbathed woman, in ragged clothes, smoothing her freshly-permanented coiffure with dirty fingernails. At this nursing home a hairdresser comes weekly.

The Nursing Home has no store or concession stand, simply a candy cart stocked and managed by the recrea-

Menu for Summer, Week I

Day 1	Day 2	Day 3	Day 4	Day 5	Day 6	Day 7
ORANGE JUICE CREAM OF WHEAT SCRAMBLED EGG TOAST MARGARINE/JELLY MILK COFF/SANKA/TEA	APPLE JUICE CHEERIOS PANCAKES/SYRUP MARGARINE MILK COFF/SANKA/TEA	CRANBERRY JUICE OATMEAL BOILED EGG TOAST/JELLY MARGARINE MILK COFF/SANKA/TEA	PINEAPPLE JUICE CORN FLAKES BANANA COFFEE CAKE MARGARINE MILK COFF/SANKA/TEA	PRUNE JUICE RICE KRISPIES FRENCH TOAST/SYRUP MARGARINE MILK COFF/SANKA/TEA	GRAPEFRUIT JUICE MAYPO SCRAMBLED EGG BLUEBERRY MUFFIN MARGARINE MILK COFF/SANKA/TEA	BLENDED JUICE PRODUCT 19 DOUGHNUT MILK COFF/SANKA/TEA
BAKED TURKEY HAM SLICE/P'APPLE RING MASHED POTATO PEAS TROPICAL FRUIT CUP BREAD/MARGARINE MILK COFF/SANKA/TEA	BRAISED BEEF CUBES ON RICE CANDIED CARROTS PLUMS BREAD/MARGARINE MILK COFF/SANKA/TEA	BREADED VEAL CUTLET SPAGHETTI/SAUCE ASPARAGUS ICE CREAM BREAD/MARGARINE MILK COFF/SANKA/TEA	TURKEY DIVAN OLD FASHIONED BREAD STUFFING CRANBERRY SAUCE JELLO/WHIPPED TOPP. ROLL/MARGARINE MILK COFF/SANKA/TEA	COUNTRY FRIED STEAK W/MUSHROOM GRAVY BAKED POTATO WAX BEANS STRAWBERRY SHORTCAKE BREAD/MARGARINE MILK COFF/SANKA/TEA	STUFFED FILET OF SOLE W/ALMONDINE SAUCE PARSLIED BAKED POTATO BUTTERED BEETS APRICOTS BREAD/MARGARINE MILK COFF/SANKA/TEA	CHICKEN CROQUETTES W/BROWN GRAVY O'BRIEN POTATO FRENCH STYLE GREEN BEANS PEARS BREAD/MARGARINE MILK COFF/SANKA/TEA
CHICKEN GUMBO SOUP/CRACKERS COLD SLICED BEEF SANDWICH LETTUCE/TOMATO MAYO SUGAR COOKIES MILK COFF/SANKA/TEA	CREAM OF TOMATO SOUP CRACKERS CHICKEN SALAD SAND. ZUCCHINI CUSTARD MILK COFF/SANKA/TEA	HOT DOGS POTATO SALAD MUSTARD/RELISH THREE BEAN SALAD MELON BREAD/MARGARINE MILK COFF/SANKA/TEA	SPLIT PEA SOUP CRACKERS TURKEY HAM SALAD SAND. W/MUSTARD POTATO CHIPS PEACHES MILK COFF/SANKA/TEA	CHICKEN & RICE SOUP CRACKERS BOLOGNA & CHEESE SAND. W/MUSTARD LETTUCE & TOMATO CHOCOLATE DROP COOKIES MILK COFF/SANKA/TEA	VEGETABLE SOUP CRACKERS FISHWICH PISTACHIO PUDDING MILK COFF/SANKA/TEA	BEEF NOODLE SOUP CRACKERS CHEESE OMLET WITH CREOLE SAUCE ORANGE & GRAPEFRUIT SECTIONS TOAST/MARGARINE MILK COFF/SANKA/TEA

tion director. Twice a year a clothing company that features easy-to-manipulate clothes (velcro closings, wide head openings, no buttons) comes to display its wares to residents.

When residents are not eating, praying, playing bingo, or at the beauty parlor, they are probably sitting. While housekeeping staff clean rooms, residents sit in the corridors. While waiting for a bath, they sit in the corridors. Before going to the dining room, they sit in the corridors. For any special event that involves moving wheelchair-bound residents, staff begin early to move people. Those moved early will sit and wait.

Some people, of course, sit simply because they cannot walk. Other people, however, sit because they have no place to go. Residents may "walk" the corridors for exercise, but unless they can find a staff member willing to help with the heavy fire doors or with the elevator, they may find their walk constricted to the one floor. Their chief destination is the dining room and occasionally, in pleasant weather, the patio, where again residents sit.

Almost every resident has a television, and the murmur of game show whistles, commercial jingles, and soap opera dialogue serves as a kind of cacophonous Muzak backdrop to the nursing home day. For some residents, television passes the time between meals, hairdresser appointments, and bingo. Other residents claim favorite shows, favorite characters, and discuss soap opera happenings among themselves. Still other residents sit and simply stare. Staff or visitors will turn on the television, presumably so the resident can stare at something; yet, though these residents ostensibly see what is happening on the small screen, they may be seeing their own inner screens and realities.

Organized outings—trips to a local park, a summer theater, or a historic village—are infrequent. The Nursing Home has no van; it charters buses for special occasions. Only a few of the residents are likely to participate in an organized outing off The Nursing Home grounds. Residents do leave The Nursing Home grounds occasionally to visit with families and frequently to visit their physicians, dentists, or optometrists. For medically-related visits, The Nursing Home will request the family to provide transportation. If the family cannot, the home will contact the state's elderly affairs department to charter its senior transportation van and send a staff aide to accompany the resident.

The home invites local Girl Scout troops, high school jazz bands, and senior citizen choruses to entertain residents. Organized theatrical or musical presentations average one per week, with up to three a week during the Christmas season. Twice a month the local Animal Rescue League brings a pet into The Nursing Home, partly to give residents a much-appreciated diversion, partly to encourage staff and visitors to adopt the animal—as occasionally happens.

The public library offers a book delivery service to city nursing home residents. A resident may request a book, which the library will deliver; or a librarian may select books from which the resident may choose. Occasionally residents of The Nursing Home use the service. The recreation director has a supply of books that residents may read. Although The Nursing Home could borrow films through a state film collective, it has no video equipment and does not do so. Some residents subscribe to a daily newspaper.

Each floor displays modified "reality orientation boards" that state the date, the names of residents whose birthday it is, and the activities planned for that day. Some nursing homes struggle to orient residents to the world beyond the nursing home's walls with exhaustive "reality orientation boards" that describe the weather, noteworthy news items, and so on. Nursing homes may also gather residents in "day rooms" for morning activities, even discussions. This home does not have "day room" activities.

The Nursing Home does not mount elaborate experiments to foster independence, such as making selected patients responsible for birds, plants, or pets; yet from fall to early spring residents from the self-care unit save bits of bread and crackers to feed the birds.

The main diversion for residents comes from outside The Nursing Home. Residents enjoy visitors, whose regular afternoon or evening stay soon becomes part of the nursing home routine, so that both staff and other residents recognize "Mrs. Smith's husband," who comes to feed her dinner; "Mr. Jones' grandchildren," who come on Sunday; or "Mrs. Medeiro's son," who brings doughnuts for the staff. Residents at The Nursing Home have lived their working lives in this factory city. Their children and grandchildren usually live within 15 miles of The Nursing Home. Indeed, the few residents who have no visitors usually have no living family. The Nursing Home encourages families to visit: staff overlook visiting hours, officially from 2 to 8, for self-care patients, whose relatives may visit whenever they wish. On Intermediate Level I and Skilled Nursing units, however, staff discourage morning and early-afternoon visits.

The Individual Adjusts

The nursing home does not replicate the individual's family home. By definition, a nursing home is a "communal" home, where residents must confront diminished personal autonomy, diminished privacy, and a diminished sense of identity.

In the world outside the nursing home, the individual routinely made an array of personal decisions, some major (where to live, whom to live with, how to spend money), some minor (what to eat, when to bathe, when to rise for breakfast). A nursing home resident makes fewer decisions. The resident need not decide when to eat, what to eat, whom to eat with, when to bathe, what to do, where to sleep, where to go, when to see the doctor, what holidays to celebrate, how to celebrate them. Nursing homes, however, vary in the autonomy allowed the individual.[5] In some nursing homes people may choose, within parameters, meals, meal times, bathing schedules, room locations, and eating companions. The Nursing Home allows little patient autonomy. Even though mealtime is the major social event, residents do not choose menus. Dietary staff interview new residents to learn their preferences and dislikes, but after that initial interview the dietary staff will set the residents' menus. Menus vary, but the staff determine the variations. Nor can patients choose mealtimes. The patient who rises early will need to wait for breakfast to be served, and the patient who sleeps late must forego breakfast. Recreational activities are so few that two are never scheduled simultaneously; hence, the resident never need choose between activities. S/he may, of course, choose not to attend a specific event; but once a concert or a performance has been arranged, staff generally insist on ensuring a resident audience for the performance. At one nursing home, when a high school concert band appeared for an evening concert, so few residents came that the band director insisted the staff marshall more of an audience. Within 10 minutes staff had rounded up about 30 residents in wheelchairs and gerichairs. Diver-

sions from routine, moreover, are so infrequent that even
a hearing-impaired resident might choose to attend a
concert.

Nor can patients usually choose rooms or roommates. Room assignments depend primarily upon the
nursing needs of the patient, the capacity of staff on
each unit, and the availability of vacant beds. The nursing
needs of the patient are the key criteria. If a resident
requires Skilled Nursing, then s/he must be on a Skilled
Nursing unit. Indeed, if a long-term resident suddenly
needs a G-tube, that requirement will by definition reclas-
sify the resident to "Skilled Nursing" status. Occasionally,
reclassification will separate a husband and wife within
the same nursing home. To increase its state-allowed census of Skilled beds, a facility in The Nursing Home's state
would need to petition the state's health department.
Room placements on Intermediate Care Levels I and II
(essentially self-care) allow staff greater discretion. Each
unit's staff, however, has its own capabilities. A spoon-fed
resident may request a room near friends, but if staff
on a unit feel they have as many "total feed" residents
as they can handle comfortably, the resident will go to
another unit. Sometimes people, particularly long-term
residents, can choose their roommate and their room,
but most room assignments are made in spite of, not
because of, resident desires. Admittedly, if a resident is
unhappy with a roommate, staff try to reassign the
patient. If the resident is a "private-paying" and not a
Medicaid resident, The Nursing Home may take individual preferences into greater account; but, again, individual preferences must coincide with nursing needs.

Perhaps as important as choice is privacy. In a congregate setting, where most rooms hold two beds, privacy

is difficult to come by. A nursing home may permit a degree of resident privacy by:

• Urging staff to knock on patients' doors and requesting permission to enter, rather than simply entering—a courtesy costing neither money nor staff time, yet permitting residents at least the illusion of control. (At The Nursing Home staff do not make it a practice to knock before entering.)

• Setting aside a number of small "visiting rooms" where a patient can comfortably visit with his or her family away from the omnipresent roommate. Roommates often become close friends, and family visitors often include the roommate in their visits; yet the resident, as well as the family, should be able to choose whether or not to include the roommate. For a modicum of privacy in the presence of a roommate unable to leave the room, families may pull the separating curtain, crowd around the single bed, and speak softly; yet if the roommate is in the windowless half of the room, daytime curtaining off can be vexatious. Also, cramped clustering around a bed doesn't promote relaxed conversation. (At The Nursing Home, residents and families go to one of the living rooms for family visits. If those are full and the first-floor conference room is available, residents and visitors may go there. If the conference room is unavailable, family and residents may use the chapel.)

• Installing private telephones, so that the resident who is physically unable to place calls at the public phone without staff assistance may have ready access to a phone. Even residents unable to dial may enjoy having regular family calls—not to mention the relief of families able to keep in touch between visits. (At The Nursing Home, residents may contract with the telephone company for private phones: 10% choose to do so. Short-term residents, who have come to The Nursing Home for specific therapy and who are expected to return to the community, may not want to arrange for a phone for their few months of residence.)

• Installing accessible public phones in a small "calling" room that would permit residents some privacy. A public phone near the nursing station, where staff and residents generally cluster, offers neither quiet nor privacy. (At The Nursing Home, the one public pay phone is on a corridor wall near the entrance.)

If patients benefit from some choice and privacy, so too patients need to retain some vestiges of their former identities. Before becoming nursing home residents, patients filled social roles: as spouse, as parent, as worker, as gardener, cook, even baseball afficionado. A humane nursing home will let the resident retain some of those mementos that will signal for him/her, as well as for other residents and staff, the nature of that "identity."[6] The Nursing Home encourages residents to bring souvenirs from their past homes, to display photographs of family members, to hang paintings, to wear their own clothes (although incontinent patients often choose to wear nursing home johnnies at night). Notwithstanding nursing home encouragement, however, residents do not truly personalize their small private space. This is partly because the private space is so small and partly because the fear of staff theft discourages families from letting patients bring valued mementos. In fact, some residents even leave wedding rings with relatives. Finally, a nursing home career often includes intermittent hospitalizations after which patients may "forfeit" space at this home and enter another nursing home—a nomadism that discourages people from bringing souvenirs.

The Care

People enter a nursing home primarily because they cannot have, in their own homes, the care they need to survive. People face an equation: on one side are their survival needs, which can range from "total care" (assistance with toileting, feeding, moving, dressing, and bathing, i.e., "activities of daily living") to assistance only with moving, or perhaps simply supervision. Indeed, "survival" itself is not clearly defined, but reflects different people's values. The requisites of survival, moreover, vary. Some care, like intravenous feeding, requires trained personnel; "custodial" care, like spoon feeding, requires only a helper. On the other side of the equation is the capability of the community home to meet the individual's needs. A person who needs minimal supervision, yet who lives alone, may need to enter a nursing home, while a person paralyzed from a stroke, yet living with a family, may remain home. Obviously, money influences the equation: individuals can buy home care resources: nurses, aides, attendants, companions. Or the larger community, through Meals-on-Wheels, subsidized home health aides, friendly visitors, and homemakers, may bolster the individual's own resources. So, too, family commitment influences the calculus: some families, quite simply, try harder and, in trying harder, succeed at meeting needs of patients that other families would find insurmountable. In the end, however, the individual confronts an inexorable equation: needs versus resources. When the individual's needs, however s/he defines them, exceed resources, the individual will eventually become a nursing home resident.

The cruel irony is that many institutions have failed, not so much to offer kindness, humanity, or meaningful choices, but simply to offer competent care. Newspaper exposes and legislative hearings have portrayed the prototypal nursing home as having filthy corridors, unkempt residents without glasses, hearing aids, and dentures, inept staff, overly-medicated patients, an absence of therapeutic regimens, theft of resident possessions, inadequate bathing facilities, sloppy pharmaceutical record-keeping, unattractive unpalatable food, and so forth. Notwithstanding the deplorable condition of some homes, people strolling through The Nursing Home, and many other nursing homes, will find immaculate corridors and dressed, kempt residents with clean fingernails and properly fitting dentures, hearing aids, and glasses. At The Nursing Home, residents are sponge-bathed daily and bathed completely an average of three times a week, although incontinent residents may be bathed three times daily.

The staff at The Nursing Home are not especially trained. At one point during my research, of day and evening clinical staff interviewed (38 full-time aides/orderlies, 4 nursing aide-coordinators, 5 charge nurses, 2 head nurses, and 1 director of nursing) (Sample A),[7] only one person—a nurse—had a bachelor's degree. The administrator has a master's degree in administration, but he has no clinical responsibilities. The home has no geriatric nurse practitioners. The absence of geriatric training, however, is not synonymous with incompetence. Most "care" required is custodial, and staff have learned to use lifts, give baths, change dressings, move and feed

patients, and make beds. Indeed, staff are more trained
than the daughters-in-law and daughters who in the community would be assuming the mantle of "caregiver"
had these patients stayed at home. As for psychosocial
care, i.e., general conversation, one writer noted that
trained nurses bent on instrumental tasks are less prone
to offer it than are housekeepers, who are not considered
"clinical" staff.[8]

Staff turnover at The Nursing Home is low, even
though salaries compare with those in other proprietary
nursing homes. In fact, an administration-sponsored survey asked The Nursing Home staff to air their complaints. Although the staff members did not need to sign
the response sheets, their responses were overwhelm-
ingly positive toward the home. The chief complaint was
wage levels. Very few staff complained about under-staffing, housekeeping support, administrative oversight, or
availability of supplies.

Staff theft, or the fear of staff theft, is a typical
nursing home problem, yet this home reports little theft
of resident or of institutional property—a statistic doubtless explained at least partially by the long tenure of
most of the staff.

The ideal number of staff remains problematic for
The Nursing Home, as for other homes that primarily
serve Medicaid patients. The state sets minimum staffing
levels so low that nursing homes with very ill patients
would be offering poor care if they did not exceed those
minimum requirements. For example, during the day
shift (7 a.m. to 3 p.m.) the state requires, for every 56-60
Skilled Nursing beds, one registered nurse, one licensed
practical nurse, and six aides. Minimum requirements
for 55-60 bed ICF I units specify two licensed practical
nurses, 5½ aides (actual requirements are in terms of

hours), and no registered nurses. ICF II regulations ask only for four aides per 46-60 beds. For evening (3 p.m. - 11 p.m.) and night (11 p.m. - 7 a.m.) shifts, the state mandates skeletal staffing: a night-time ICF II unit of 46-60 beds needs only two aides to meet state requirements. Even the Skilled Nursing unit at night needs only one registered nurse and four aides for 56-60 beds. The Nursing Home argues that low Medicaid payments ($58 per day per patient) discourage the hiring of additional staff. Nevertheless, on most shifts on most days, The Nursing Home exceeds state requirements.

For Medicare patients, the home contracts with a private agency to provide physical therapy according to physician prescriptions. The state's law does not require nursing homes to offer physical therapy for non-Medicare residents. For non-Medicare residents, staff aides offer "gate training" and "range of motion" therapy, according to physician orders. Three to five times weekly the recreation director offers "aerobic chair exercises" for interested residents. For Medicare residents needing speech therapy, the nursing home will similarly contract with a private agency. For non-Medicare patients, however, the home offers no speech therapy analogous to "gate training" or "range of motion" physical therapy. A pharmaceutical consultant reviews patient medication orders regularly. The home has no occupational therapist. The home does have a social worker who, in addition to processing admissions, does "psychosocial histories," as required by state regulations, and attempts to keep in touch with resident families. In 1985 The Nursing Home instituted its first family support group, run by the social worker, who invites speakers from the community (a hospice physician, for instance). In time, families may use the support group as an advocacy organization as well as a way of alleviating their combination of tension/guilt/anguish. Until that happens though, families generally siphon complaints through the social worker.

In terms of care, a key failing of The Nursing Home, as of most American nursing homes, is what one writer[9] called "the absent physician." Families do not abandon relatives when they enter a nursing home, but often the family physician does. If a family physician refuses to treat a patient in The Nursing Home, the family may choose a different physician. If a family cannot or will not choose another physician, the resident may be assigned to the private practice of the community physician who serves on retainer as the medical director of the nursing home. Even if a physician continues to treat a patient once s/he enters a nursing home, however, that care may be sporadic, limited to fleeting visits and occasional phone directives. Medicaid regulations require a physician to see an ICF patient once every 60 days—hardly an ongoing relationship; yet staff here and elsewhere complain of the "invisible physician" who visits only to sign required forms and wave hello to his patients. When a patient needs a change in regimen or medications, staff frequently have to make repeated telephone calls to the physician. If the patient's physician cannot be contacted and staff believe the patient needs medical attention, the resident will be sent to the emergency room of a nearby hospital.

The Patients

Every resident has confronted the equation of needs versus resources. In this nursing home, residents' needs far outweigh resources.

The prototypical resident in The Nursing Home is an 83-year-old widow who has lived in the home 18 months.

Before coming to The Nursing Home, 45% of the residents (from Sample B) lived in their own homes, 19% lived with children, and 35% lived in a different long-term care institution. Most residents, even those who lived alone, have family. See Table 2.1 for patient profile.

One author noted that "the unfittest survive."[10] A walk through this nursing home supports that contention. An elderly person's confusion often propels families to seek nursing home care. According to the judgment of both the social worker and a head nurse at The Nursing Home, at admission 51% of patients recognized who they were, where they were, and who their visitors were all or most of the time, 21% were lucid some of the time, and 28% were rarely or never lucid.

Most residents had limited mobility. Only 35% of residents could walk unassisted, 8% needed a walker, 4% needed a cane, 29% needed a wheelchair, 6% a gerichair, and 17% were bed-to-chair. Six percent of residents were legally blind; 15% had impaired hearing. Twenty-six percent could not speak intelligibly. Twenty-four percent could not eat unassisted. Even the comparatively "independent" residents, however, may have seemed to be so only in comparison with their nursing home counterparts. For instance, a resident who could walk the corridors unassisted might not have been strong enough or steady enough to go for a walk outside.

Residents, however, are more than the sum of their physical disabilities. Each resident has brought a unique history to The Nursing Home. In the midst of grave illness and deterioration it is easy to overlook the people themselves. Residents' lives echo common themes, such as:

• A worklife spent in nearby textile mills or jewelry

Table 2.1.   Patient Profile. (N - 145; Sample B)

		Number
Sex:	Male	27
	Female	118
Marital Status:	Married	14
	Widowed	92
	Separated/Divorced	10
	Never Married	29
Religion:	Catholic	103
	Protestant	37
	Orthodox	4
	Unknown	1
Prior Occupation:	At Home	12
	Unskilled Factory Work	98
	Retail/Office	22
	Professional/Self-Employed	12
	Unknown	1
Ethnicity:	Irish	26
	English/Scottish	38
	French	44
	Italian	13
	Portuguese	6
	Other	18
Preadmission Residence:	Own Home	66
	Child's Home	28
	Other Institution	50
	Unknown	1
Lucidity:	Judged Lucid	74
	Judged Sometimes Lucid	31
	Judged Rarely/Never Lucid	40
Living Family:	Spouse	15
	Child(ren)	93
	Sibling	56
Mobility:	Bed-to-Chair	25
	Gerichair	8
	Wheelchair	43
	Walker/Cane	18
	Walks Unassisted	51
Physical Limitations:	Cannot Eat Unassisted	110
	Cannot Speak Intelligibly	108
	Legally Blind	9
	Hearing Impaired	15
	Deaf	7
Tenure in Nursing Home:	Months Median	37
	Months Maximum	69
Age:	Years Median	83.5

factories. A young woman might have immigrated to the United States from Italy or Canada right before the first World War, found a job in a mill, left to marry and have children, and returned intermittently to the mill. Most worked as unskilled or semi-skilled laborers in factories employing scores of their counterparts.

• Domesticity. Women who never married were devoted daughters, aunts, siblings. Only a few of the female residents had held jobs that could be considered "professional." Several women had been registered nurses or schoolteachers, but even these women might not have called their occupations "careers" with all the connotations that "career" holds for today's employed woman.

• Bereavement. Nursing home residents have inevitably lived longer than most of the people they have known and loved, and feel a concomitant sense of loss. Social work histories tell of the spouses, children, and siblings who have died. One gerontologist[11] sought to compare nursing home residents with friends still in the community. When he asked residents to identify community friends, however, most could not. So, too, these nursing home residents have lost many of the people who loved and supported them throughout their lives.

• Isolation from the larger cultural/political community. Most of the residents of The Nursing Home were never politically nor culturally active. They spent their lives working in factories, raising children, participating in church activities, making friends. Not surprisingly, then, the dearth of political/cultural activities available in the nursing home does not distress them. For instance, many residents never went to the library while living in the community. Now that they are "institutionalized," they have not developed a new-found interest in reading. Hence, few residents use the library's "homebound" service. The home does not subscribe to magazines for residents, but, then, most residents did not subscribe to magazines when they lived in the community. The nursing home does not pipe Vivaldi into the dining room during meals—but most residents were never lovers of classical music.

   • Blue-collar incomes. Most residents were not impoverished. They had earned enough in the mills to raise families, furnish apartments and take small vacations without depending on welfare, but, conversely, most residents had lived modestly while they were employed and even more modestly once they needed to depend upon Social Security. Jewelry factories and textile mills generally do not give pensions to Depression-era employees.

A Lament for a Lost Home

If all the people who evaluate nursing homes—the academicians, the gerontologists, and bureaucrats, in addition to the nonelderly "public"—were to recite the accoutrements of an ideal "home," they would probably include comfortable chairs clustered around a fireplace, carpets, paintings, music, cases bulging with books, plants, a garden, colorful upholstery, sunshine, a place to share coffee with a friend. The Nursing Home has vinyl floors and upholstery, mauve still lifes on the walls, heavy drapes, no fireplace, very few comfortable chairs, no stereo, no bookcases, no garden, and no pleasant intimate spots for conversation.

   The Nursing Home, like most of its counterparts, does not look like a family home in part because of governmental supervision. Thirty years ago many nursing homes and rest homes offered "homey" rooms, with carpets, plants, paintings, books, and home-style meals, all in a "real" house in a residential neighborhood in an older section of town. The "real" house looked and felt homey. Staff consisted of an elderly widow (who may have been a registered nurse) or an older couple, committed to offering warmth and security and supervision and meals. They may or may not have supplemented their own labor with a cleaning woman.

Nostalgic recollections of house-based "rest homes" feature an optimum combination of warm caregivers, mildly incapacitated residents, and suitable facilities. But, although caregivers could be warm matronly souls, they might also be mercenary women scheming to profit from an essentially helpless clientele. Similarly, these homes did not necessarily provide physical therapy, intravenous feeding, or feeding-tubes, nor could they comfortably accommodate severely demented patients, incontinent patients, or comatose patients. The homey home did not offer smoke detectors, sprinkler systems, alarm systems hooked into local fire stations, fire doors, easy exit points, and nonflammable construction. Stringent fire regulations forced many of the "mom and pop" nursing homes out of business.

Benign governmental legislation assaulted nursing homes with a barrage of regulations and specifications and inspections. And because funding and jurisdiction for nursing homes fell under the "hospital" arm of HEW, not the social service one, the regulations, specifications, and inspections hark back to those appropriate for a strictly medical facility.[12] Thus, a nursing home must have heavy fire doors, sprinklers, at least minimally-credentialled staff, and admission and discharge forms. And investigators investigate, not the quality of life, however that might be defined, but record-keeping, cleanliness, kitchen facilities, physician signatures, levels of care, and staffing levels. Investigators, in short, use quasi-hospital criteria to evaluate the nursing home, asking, not how warm a home it is, but how medically sufficient it is. Not surprisingly, many of the "homey" facilities of the past died under the barrage of governmental regulation.

Nostalgia for these preregulatory rest homes, though, is misplaced. The Nursing Home only partly reflects governmental regulations. The home also reflects the patients themselves. The food, for instance, is bland; yet the constraints on food preparation might stymie L'Escoffier. The Nursing Home must serve nutritious food that is palatable to people who are limited to special diets, who have pronounced likes and dislikes, and who represent different ethnic backgrounds. At this nursing home many residents have sugar and/or sodium and/or cholesterol-restricted diets. Still other residents cannot chew. Reflecting a range of culinary lifestyles, residents have pronounced opinions on "good" food: some residents consider pasta essential; others want meat-and-potatoes; still others enjoy pastry and coffee. Nutritional value notwithstanding, many of the residents at this home spurn fresh fruits and vegetables, preferring the canned variety.

Some of the "institutional" features, however bleak, enhance patients' well-being. While vinyl floors evoke hospital corridors, carpets impede wheelchairs and walkers, as well as retain odors from incontinent patients' accidents. Chairs upholstered in colorful chintz fabrics brighten a living room, but incontinent patients would be reluctant to use them. Metal hospital beds facilitate patient maneuvers. Nursing station call buttons let the patient contact a staff member quickly. People in wheelchairs and walkers need large elevators, not elegant circular stairways.

Indeed, prototypical designs for nursing homes of the future look even less "homey." Closed monitor video screens with intercoms in patients' rooms—reminiscent of Big Brother—would let staff quickly communicate with a patient requesting assistance. Closed circuit television would permit staff greater flexibility in allowing confused patients simply to "wander." Circularly designed patient units, with the nursing station in the center of a ring of patient rooms, would similarly facilitate staff supervision. Currently, some gerontological researchers[13] are working to develop robots capable of serving as patient aides; for instance, a robot might deliver a glass of water to a thirsty resident. Sliding doors that open automatically, beds that patients can regulate themselves, video-telephones—all may be standard in the nursing home of the future, yet such technologically-inspired improvements will not yield a homey structure.

This book purports to describe the nursing home from a family paradigm, to suggest the extent to which an institutional "home" can provide friendship, warmth, and dignity; yet the *mise en scene* is wrong. The home's fire doors, small rooms, concrete patio, fixed schedules, and bland walls do not evoke "home." Janet Tulloch, a nursing home resident with cerebral palsy, lamented that "A Home is not a Home" in a participant-observation study of her nursing home.[14] More accurately, "A nursing home is not a house." The nursing home does not look like a house, yet the key question is, "Can a sterile facility that seems like a combination hospital-motel still offer the requisites of a home?" Or, more succinctly, can a home exist apart from a house?

Images of home are invariably tied to images of a

house; and "house" carries with it emotional connotations. All people, however, will not conjure up the same images or the same emotional responses.

Visitors strolling through The Nursing Home may be envisioning it as their future home, and wondering how they will feel in such an institutional facility, what amenities they will want, what indignities they would find insufferable. They may be imagining their reactions to the plaster Madonna lifted onto a dining room table, the omnipresent chatter of staff, the corridors, the dearth of music, the lack of books, the monotonous routine, the lack of movies, the banality of meals. We gaze through the lenses of our own experiences and expectations.

The residents of this nursing home, however, are not the same people as those strolling down the corridors. Many residents are in wheelchairs or walkers. Some are virtually bed-ridden. Some are so confused that they think they are 20-year-old brides preparing meals, not 85-year-old widows in a nursing home. These residents' images of "home" may not feature the same accoutrements as the homes of the able-bodied, nonelderly spectators. Many residents have come to The Nursing Home from solitary third-floor apartments from which they rarely ventured forth because they feared neighborhood muggers. While contemporary onlookers might value art, music, books, and flowers in a home, these residents might value elevators, cleanliness, regular meals, safety, warmth. Omnipresent roommates and bustling staff may not seem intrusive presences, but welcome companions. Unlike the nonelderly professionals who evaluate geriatric long-term care options, these nursing home residents are an average of 83 years old, are veterans of harsh working lives, have survived children, spouses, and friends, and have moved to a nursing home, not because they yearned to live in an institution, but because their community home—their "true" home—could not sufficiently meet their needs for survival. These nursing home residents may not find the "institution" so grim a home.

Chapter 3

A Home of Friends

*What life have you if you have not life together? There is no life
that is not in community—T.S. Eliot*[1]

The search for a familial community within a nursing
home demands persistence. The physical trappings of
the facility point to an institution; staff dress like institutional staff; residents follow an institutionally-prescribed
routine. The most familial aspect of a nursing home is
the word "home," which at times seems an ironic mis-
nomer.

The search for a community begins with the residents themselves. In a community people bond with one
another. Empathizing with each other, they will find at
least one other person to talk to, to feel comfortable
with, to confide in—in short, a friend. In an institution
(as defined by Goffman), on the other hand, the individual, treated like an object, becomes one; and people
cease to empathize, to share, to trust each other as they
become, simply, "inmates." Although inmates live in con-
fined, even cramped, quarters, they remain emotionally
isolated. Friendships provide one major test of the "in-

stitutionality" of a nursing home. If residents form no friendships, then the home, contrary to its optimistic nomenclature, is as institutional a setting as Goffman's asylum. If residents make friends, however, then the setting does not squelch the very human needs of people to connect with other people.

A nursing home may seem an unlikely spot for friendships. People playing a word association game would hardly associate "nursing home" with "camaraderie," "companionship," or "friend." They would imagine a friendless place where people stare forlornly into space, waiting for visitors. Indeed, the play, *The Gin Game*,[2] reflects the popular image of the nursing home as a social wasteland. In the play two nursing home residents, a divorced man and a widow, sit bickering with one another, trying to decide whether or not to play cards, as they wait for the visitors who will not come. Around them their fellow residents sit, also waiting for visitors. Goffman would recognize the nursing home of *The Gin Game* as a classic institution.

Physically, The Nursing Home, like most other nursing homes, presents barriers to patient movement. Heavy fire doors between wings, elevators with inaccessible controls, a paucity of visiting spaces—all limit resident movement to one floor, if not one wing of one floor.

The emotional atmosphere of nursing homes is distinctly unconvivial. In a place where many residents leave, often to die in a hospital, less often to transfer to another nursing home, even more rarely to go home, every resident recognizes that friendship may be short-lived. Furthermore, the fact of impending death may encourage residents to turn inward, rather than reach out to others.[3]

The patient role[4] itself precludes reaching out. Residents who enter a nursing home for a prescribed therapeutic regimen, such as physical therapy after a hip replacement or recuperation after a colostomy, are looking, not to establish friendships within this new community, but simply to recuperate enough to leave. Other residents, those not slated to go home, may be too ill to spend time and/or energy seeking out new friends.[5]

Some residents are confused. Others are depressed. Still others are deranged. Often families that are able to cope with parental incontinence balk at coping with parental confusion, and confused residents find themselves in nursing homes, where they are no more likely to establish meaningful relationships than they were in their family homes. Lucid residents living beside deranged residents may grow depressed[6] as they recognize that competence is not necessarily an asset within the nursing home.

In the world outside the nursing home people befriend co-workers, neighbors, friends of friends, fellow sporting or gardening or cooking enthusiasts, classmates. Friendships tend to be class-based. You befriend people whom you regularly meet, and you regularly meet people from the same social milieu. Even when people from different social classes mingle, the invisible Maginot Line of class usually intrudes to cement people within their own niches.

A nursing home is a virtually classless society, where vestiges of class are all but invisible. People are assigned to units according to their nursing needs, not their income or social class. Indeed, within a given nursing home residents are generally unable to "buy" better accommodations or better food; and even if they could, the costs of nursing home care are so high that almost everybody in time depends upon Medicaid.[7] Walls and bureau space allow little room to display items that might illuminate a resident's past life. Although women may wear jewelry within the nursing home, most leave precious jewels with families. Even ethnicity remains muted in nursing homes, where staff address residents by their first names. Physicians, lawyers, bricklayers, housewives, servants, prostitutes, mill workers—the common denominator for nursing home residence is age and disability. Within a nursing home the mill owner may easily sit beside the mill worker. Past occupation is neither salient nor obvious.

A nursing home, however, offers residents one thing essential for friendships: time. Despite architectural and emotional barriers, conviviality exists. In the dreariest nursing homes some residents make friends.[8] In fact, some people—"expanders"—have more friends in the nursing home than they had in the community.[9] Residents have days and evenings full of leisure time—no tasks, no jobs, no responsibilities for self-care, no family obligations, no bookkeeping chores, no housekeeping needs. With nothing to do and no place to go, residents sit and talk to each other. Indeed, the role of friend is the one nonpatient role left to nursing home residents. A woman may no longer be a gardener, a cook, or a seamstress. Nor is she a spouse, a parent, or a sibling because over time even familial relationships degenerate into visitor and visitee. A man is no longer a machinist or a physician or a carpenter or a husband. The major role open to nursing home residents is that of patient, an essentially passive role, where the resident follows a prescribed therapeutic regimen and obeys staff instructions. Intimacy, however, remains a critical human need[10]; and residents who find friends are not so desolate as *Gin Game* characters.[11]

Searching for Friends

Josephine S., Helen T., John J., Jim S., Eva W.—they offer

solid evidence of friendships. Seeing rows of wheelchairs lining the walls, the casual visitor to The Nursing Home may overlook Josephine and Helen and John and Jim and Eva, but the persistent visitor soon recognizes the cliques, the partners, the patterned seating for meals and rosary and bingo. In patient rooms the omnipresent observer will see roommates comfortably reminiscing with each other, discussing each other's families, enjoying each other's visitors.

Sitting in a straight-backed chair, Josephine S. reads aloud. She used to be a nurse in a state hospital. Now an 81-year-old widow, she has one divorced daughter who lives alone with a teenage son. Because Josephine has Alzheimer's disease, she remembers neither the nursing job, the daughter, nor the grandson. She does remember how to read, however; and her ever-present companion, a Portuguese widower who understands no English, sits by her side, listening to her lilting intonations of a language neither she nor he comprehends. In the morning he looks for her. When she sees him, she finds a book and reads. At meals they sit together.

Eva W. reminisces about her "fast" life: many men, many friends, many parties. Now 83, she is the nursing home's social butterfly, welcoming new residents, helping confused ones, joining in a close friend's birthday celebration, gossiping with everybody. In pleasant weather she walks slowly outside, encouraging a walker-bound friend who is afraid to venture forth alone.

Jim S., an amputee, has found a fellow baseball aficionado in the nursing home. Together they sit in their wheelchairs outside the back entrance overlooking the parking lot listening to the Boston Red Sox lose yet another game.

Helen T., a 95-year-old widow, and John J., a widower in his late 70s, used to sit together regularly when they lived on the same first floor unit. When Helen became ill and moved to a more intensive nursing unit on the second floor, John would go upstairs and escort her to bingo games and concerts and holiday parties. Now she is better and is again on John's unit.

Annunziata G. and Margaret M., two retired nurses, have shared the same room for four years. When one went to the hospital for a short stay, the other sent her a card every day. When Margaret, a diabetic, cheats on her diet by eating ice cream surreptitiously in the bathroom, Annunziata covers for her. When Annunziata's family takes her for a family outing to their home or a restaurant, they include Margaret. One taught the other how to knit an afghan.

In this nursing home, some residents have made friends. Josephine S., Annunziata G., Helen T., Eva W., Jim S.—they have found, if not soul mates, at least amiable companions. The evidence of bonds between residents bespeaks a community beneath the institutional facade of the nursing home—but people like Josephine, Annunziata, Helen, Eva, and Jim do not predominate. Onlookers will also see people staring morosely at the walls, sitting beside each other, yet oblivious to the people around them—characters lifted straight from *The Gin Game*. Some residents silently await meals, baths, and the changing of bed linen without acknowledging the companions who wait with them.

Sociological Tools

Observation and anecdotes provide insight into nursing home life, but the tools of a sociologist may help even more in the search for a community. A sociologist by definition studies groups of people. S/he looks for interaction among and between groups, patterns of interaction, and "facts," not about individuals, but about groups. Because a sociologist is concerned with groups, sociological tools involve analysis, often by computer, of aggregate data from many individuals. Those techniques may reveal facets of a community that the institutional decor of the nursing home masks.

Clearly, The Nursing Home has residents who have made friends, as well as residents who have remained "loners." A key question is: How pervasive are those friendships? Even in the most Kafkaesque institution, a few people may be fortunate enough to find sympathetic fellow inmates, while in many "communities" some individuals remain isolated. We know that bonds between some residents exist in The Nursing Home, but we need to know how pervasive those bonds are. Sociological techniques can address that question.

The Pervasiveness of Friendships

"Friend" is an imprecise term, connoting sharing, intimacy, companionship, loyalty, and trust. One person's friend may be another person's acquaintance and another's companion. People's criteria for friendship vary. Some friends see each other regularly. Some may share intimate confidences. Others who consider themselves friends may simply exchange holiday cards.

To define "friends" in this nursing home, I used a behavioral definition: People who sat together regularly, ate together, and watched television together were considered "friends." To determine the friendship networks of nursing home residents, I asked unit staff to identify each resident's regular companions. Staff were chosen because they, unlike outside observers, know the social ambiance of their unit—who likes whom, who is feuding with whom, who serves as mediator, who belongs to what clique, who has recently lost a good friend. If staff disagreed about a particular relationship, I judged that it was not strong enough to constitute a friendship bond. From staff on each unit, I constructed a consensual portrait of interaction that identified for each resident the number of friends, from 0 to 6.

The disadvantage of this behavioral snapshot of interaction is that it may overstate the intensity with which people regard their companions. People who regularly talk with each other may feel they are pleasant acquaintances, but not truly friends. One common technique of judging friendship uses a resident questionnaire[12] that asks each person whom he considers a friend, whom he confides in, and with whom he feels most comfortable. In a nursing home that kind of questionnaire has limitations. Many residents cannot respond to oral or written questions. Some people cannot hear, see, speak, write; or, if they can, may not understand a questionnaire enough to respond dependably. Still other people might not choose to answer. In *Assessing the Elderly,* Kane and Kane[13] describe the dilemmas of researchers determined to assess mental competence. Any construction of social life that relied on resident questionnaires would have to restrict the portrait to residents physically and mentally able, as well as willing, to respond. Although such residents may in fact be the ones who have made friends, a study of friendships need not begin with that bias.

Also, a snapshot of interaction may overstate the number of loners. Residents new to The Nursing Home may not yet have had time to make friends, while veterans of the home may have recently lost a friend. The turnover of nursing home residents is considerable as residents die, transfer, or return home. Long-standing friendships often end abruptly. This one-time portrait will show both newcomers and veterans as "loners" where a later or an earlier portrait might show that, in fact, they were not.

At The Nursing Home, the snapshots of interaction belie the notion of institutional aloofness. At one given time, the research covered 145 residents (Sample B).[14] Fifty-two had no friends. The median number of friends was 1; the maximum, 6. Indeed, the portraits of interaction are complex, showing cliques, dyads, and extraordinarily sociable individuals who managed to befriend even relative "loners." Figure 3.1 diagrams the interaction on one of the nursing home's four units.

Sociable residents—the nursing home's own social-ites—stand out in the diagrams of interaction. Their backgrounds are diverse, yet they have a love of people and an ability to forge bonds with others, even in the most unlikely setting of a nursing home. Eva W. is one. She spends her days as an unofficial friendly visitor. She greets new visitors, tells them about the people and staff on their unit, and introduces them to other residents. If a resident is sad, Eva will try to cheer her. If a resident is reluctant to walk, Eva will walk with her, although Eva herself walks

Figure 3.1. Friendship Patterns—Unit West I. (N = 47; Sample B)

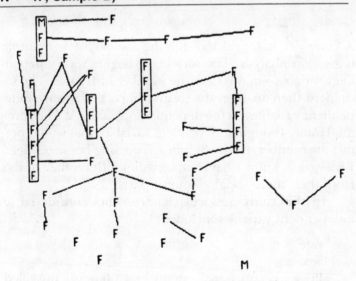

gingerly. The mailman, the social worker, the desk receptionist—all smile when she approaches. She has befriended
confused residents, depressed residents, and disgruntled
residents. Her family consists of a daughter who is unable
to visit regularly. Her husbands, siblings, and friends have
all died. Nevertheless, her love for people has helped her
transform the nursing home, her final home, into a surrogate family, where residents and staff are friends.

Compilation of "friendship" diagrams suggests the
nursing home has some features of a community, yet this
evidence is not sufficient. Many residents admittedly have
made friends. West 1, the unit shown in Figure 3.1, is a
"self-care" unit. On West 1, the loners are a small minority;
but in The Nursing Home as a whole many residents—35%
of the total—have no friends. They emerge as loners who,
notwithstanding the closeness of congregate living, have
remained emotionally isolated from their fellow residents.
The persistence of these loners deserves investigation. Who
are the loners? Why do they remain isolated?

Loners

A common statistical tool for the sociologist is multiple
regression analysis. The sociologist begins with a dependent variable—in this case, the number of friends. The sociologist then analyzes the relative impact of diverse independent variables on the dependent variable. At The Nursing Home, I sought independent variables that would predict the number of friends for each nursing home resident.
I wanted to know what characteristics differentiate loners
from their more sociable counterparts.

In this study, resident characteristics considered as
independent variables included:

Age
Sex
Prior occupational status (at home, unskilled,

skilled, professional)

Tenure within the nursing home (measured in number of months since initial admission, regardless of intermittent hospitalizations)

Preadmission residence (a categorical "dummy" dichotomous variable, indicating whether the resident had lived in the community or in another institution)

Family ties

1. Dummy dichotomous variables, coded as the presence of a living spouse, sibling, or child. Theoretically, relatives could be delineated as visiting or nonvisiting relatives; but in fact most relatives lived nearby and visited at least occasionally

2. Frequency of visits: a scale created for each resident by coding the frequency of visits from different visitors

Lucidity (the social worker evaluated the lucidity of residents as: never/rarely lucid, sometimes lucid; usually lucid. The criterion was the resident's ability to recognize her surroundings and her family visitors)

Physical limitations, specifically:

1. Ability to speak (a dichotomous variable: resident could speak or could not)

2. Ability to eat unassisted (another dichotomous variable: resident could eat unassisted or could not. This variable was considered important because the dining room is the major social center)

3. Ability to see (resident was legally blind or not)

4. Ability to hear (a three-part scale, from deaf, to hearing-impaired, to hearing)

5. Mobility (a scale of mobility, ranging from bed-to-chair, to gerichair, to wheelchair, to

walker, walks assisted only with cane, walks unassisted)

Again, the goal of multiple regression analysis was to identify independent variables whose effect on sociability could be considered "significant." A regression equation takes the form,

$$Y = ax_1 + bx_2 + cx_3 + dx_4 + ex_5 + fx_6 + gx_n.$$

Y represents the dependent variable; x, the various independent variables. Each independent variable has a coefficient, based on the standard deviations of that variable. The coefficient (a,b,c,d, and so forth) represents the strength of the relationship between the two variables, independent and dependent. The value of that coefficient, also known as a beta, can range from .00 (no relationship) to (+) or (−) .99 (the strongest relationship). A negative beta points to an inverse relationship between two interval-level variables. A negative beta between income and age, for instance, would signify that as people grow older, their income shrinks. A positive beta points to a direct relationship: as people age, their income increases. Multiple regression equations allow the researcher to investigate the impact of many independent variables upon one dependent variable. Such equations permit the researcher to focus on the individual effects of one independent variable, while holding constant the other independent variables. More specifically, the comparison of betas permits judgments about the relative strength of different predictive variables.

Each regression equation, moreover, has a value labelled as R^2. R^2 represents that proportion of the variance in the dependent variable that is explained by the independent variables. For instance, an R^2 of .75 means that 75% of the variance in the dependent variable, Y, was explained by the various independent variables (Xes). In contrast, a regression equation with an R^2 of .15 is far weaker: in that equation, the independent variables explained only 15% of the variation in Y. The proportion of the variance that the equation does not explain is the error term. A high error term (and, concomitantly, a low R^2) indicates that the model put forth by the equation may have omitted a key variable or variables.

Two regression equations were constructed. In the first equation, the existence of friends was a dummy dependent variable (the Y); that is, a resident had no friends or had at least one friend. A dummy variable permits a dichotomous coding of information: yes/no. In this case, each resident was coded as a "loner" or not. That dependent variable, which delineated social isolation from community, was called "friendship." In the second equation, the actual number of friends—from 0 to 6—was the dependent variable. In a sense, the computer was asking, "What people are likely to be loners? What people are likely to join into the nursing home-as-community? What people are likely to have more friends within the nursing home?"

The computer's response was clear. As Table 3.1 shows, lucid, sighted residents who could speak were more likely to enter into the community of the nursing home. Or, from a different perspective, confused, aphasic, and blind residents were likely to be loners. Friendship implies an ability to communicate. When confusion, aphasia, or blindness blocks communication, that person will be unable to forge strong bonds with companions.

Age *per se* proved no deterrent to friendships. Older people were no more likely to be isolated than younger ones. Nor did mobility—so important outside the nursing home—influence sociability within the nursing home. Residents were rated on a mobility scale: from bedridden to a geri-chair to a wheelchair to a walker to a cane to independent. Independent residents were no more isolated than wheelchair-bound residents. Indeed, the unimpor-

Table 3.1.   Regression Analysis, Considering Friendship and Number of Friends as the Dependent Variables and Resident Characteristics as the Independent Variables. (N = 145; Sample B)

Resident Characteristics	Friendship Beta	Number of Friends Beta
Sex	-.02	.04
Age	.00	-.07
Prior Occupational Status	-.10	-.11
Tenure in The Nursing Home	-.11	-.21*
Preadmission Residence	.01	-.13
Family Ties		
A Living Spouse	-.07	.03
A Living Child	-.09	-.12
A Living Sibling	-.02	.05
Frequency of Visits	.05	.06
Lucidity	.23*	.25*
Physical Limitations		
Able to Speak	.25*	.21*
Able to Eat Without Assistance	.12	.08
Able to See	.24*	.17*
Able to Hear	.09	.11
Mobility	.03	.05
R^2 =	.37	.39

level of significance
*p .001

tance of limited mobility within the nursing home marks a sharp contrast with the restricted lives of wheelchair-bound people in the larger community.

Tenure within The Nursing Home did not affect the *formation* of friendships: long-term residents were not more likely to be friendless than their shorter-term counterparts.

Tenure did affect the *number* of friends, however. The negative beta (-.21) suggests an inverse relationship: as tenure in The Nursing Home increased, the number of friends decreased. Veterans of this nursing home were likely to have a smaller circle of friends, perhaps because long-term residents had lost friends through death or transfer.

One would think that residents with strong ties to the world outside the nursing home should not need to establish friendships within the nursing home as much as people whose community ties are weaker. Accordingly, I hypothesized that 1) residents with living spouses, children, and siblings, and 2) residents with frequent visitors would be less likely to make friends than residents without living relatives. Similarly, I hypothesized that residents admitted to The Nursing Home directly from the community, rather than from another nursing home, would not feel so strong a need to reach out to their fellow residents. The data supported neither hypothesis. The existence of living family members had no impact upon friendships, and the person's preadmission residence also had no impact.

The R^2 of the equation where "friendship" was the dependent variable is .37; the R^2 of the equation with the number of friends as the dependent variable is .39. In other words, residents' physical limitations explain just under 40% of the variance in both models of friendship formation—a strong predictive model from a social scientist's vantage.

Some residents made no friends within The Nursing Home simply because of their limited ability to forge bonds with others. Indeed, a very confused person might live a detached, solitary existence even in the midst of a loving family. The patient with Alzheimer's disease probably retreated from friends and family long before entering the nursing home. Since friendship depends upon communication, and since people usually communicate through

speech, the aphasic resident may well remain socially isolated, regardless of the setting. Many of the residents who
stared aloofly into space did so because they simply could
not reach out to those around them, not because the institutional trappings of this nursing home stifled their ability
to empathize.

Blind residents may be the only ones who suffer more
restricted social lives in a nursing home than in the community. A blind person accustomed to a home and friends
may not so easily re-establish that comfortable sense of
familiarity in a new setting. If the new setting is a nursing
home, moreover, staff fearful that the blind resident may
fall or bump into an object may unduly restrict the individual's movements. Positioned in a room or a chair, the
blind person—no matter how lucid and how eager for
friendship—may easily find him- or herself trapped in a
solitary world.

Clarice B. is blind, and her life at The Nursing Home
bespeaks the grim existence of a person unfamiliar with
her surroundings, fearful of exploring a new home, surrounded by strangers, and frightened of the strange
sounds and movements in this dark world. Staff, moreover,
admit to an anxiety about her. They do not encourage her
to walk and meet people. Indeed, The Nursing Home is
reluctant to admit blind people. Clarice spends her days
yelling, weeping, demanding staff attention, complaining,
and weeping more. She refuses to go to the dining room
for meals. In discussing "unfavorite" patients, many staff
ranked her near the top and said they would be pleased
if she left this nursing home for another one.

Other "loners," however, are isolated because they simply cannot communicate. Two comatose patients understandably have no friends. One man suffering from alcoholism and cirrhosis of the liver behaves erratically, alternately thrashing out at staff and ignoring staff. He has no
friends among the residents. Harriet O. also has no friends

in The Nursing Home. She was labelled retarded as a young child, lived in a state institution throughout most of her childhood and adolescence, then returned home to her mother when the state forged ahead with deinstitutionalization of state facilities. When her widowed mother died, Harriet had no convenient potential caregivers—no siblings, no father, no caring extended family. She came by default to this nursing home, where she has not yet spoken.

A few people are uninterested in friendships. Patricia Y. is a wealthy, 83-year-old, never-married woman. The daughter of a local industrialist, she lived a life that revolved around travel. She has no friends or family. For the last ten years she has hired a live-in companion; and even now that she lives in a nursing home, she continues to pay the companion a retainer. The companion visits daily. The resident does not leave her room, even for meals.

Two findings stand out. First, friendships do exist within the nursing home. Second, people likely to emerge as loners suffer from mental and physical limitations that impede communication.

The nursing home begins to resemble a community. The community, however, is one with no glaring clues to residents' income, social class, education, occupation, family history, or ethnicity. In short, the factors so important to friendships in the world outside the nursing home are muted within the nursing home.

Classless Friendships

To understand possible common bonds between residents, this research investigated similarities that friendship partners shared. Did they have the same religion? Did they work at the same occupation? Were both widowers or bachelors or spinsters or widows? Did both have children? Did both represent the same ethnic backgrounds? Did women befriend only women and men befriend only men? Or did the nursing home environment itself shape friendships? Much as in a school, did residents' varying tenure represent a potential bond; that is, did veterans of the home cluster together? Or was room location the key to friendships?

The results (Table 3.2) suggest two areas in common, one surprising, the other expected. Of 110 friendship-dyads, 87% lived on the same unit—a result substantiated by other studies of nursing home life.[15] Since friendships depend a great deal upon the frequency with which people interact, and since residents on the same unit will inevitably interact most with each other insomuch as they eat together, watch each other's visitors, and sit in the same corridors, unit location as the basis for friendship was not surprising.

The surprising finding is the bond of contemporaneous age. For the purposes of this study, contemporaries were defined as people born within 10 years of each other (a distinction used by Chappell).[16] Although "the elderly," especially the disabled elderly, may seem a monolithic block, contemporaries did in fact search each other out. They remembered the same political heroes, the same critical sports games, the same world catastrophes. Furthermore, they remembered the Depression, World War II, and the Korean war from the same demographic vantage. When they talked to each other, they understood each other's vocabulary.

Ethnicity was comparatively unimportant. The sociological literature portrays ethnicity as a key social cleavage that shows itself not only in voting behavior, but in residential communities. These residents' friendships did not reflect ethnic identities. New England enjoys a wealth of immigrant communities. Perhaps residents living in so polyglot an area had long since learned to appreciate people from different cultures; or perhaps ethnicity itself is so muted in the nursing home, especially in a facility

where staff call residents by their first names, that residents
no longer considered ethnic background an important
bond for friends.

Table 3.2 shows only demographic bonds that can
easily be established—the structural variables that predominate in sociological research. Some of the friendships, however, reflect a helping-helper bond. One woman needed
help walking; her friend would walk with her. One man
would push the wheelchair of another resident. One lucid
resident would regularly visit a sometimes-confused neigh-
bor; and, although the confused resident may or may not
have enjoyed the regular visits, the visitor clearly enjoyed
helping her friend. With a very busy staff and one social
worker, this nursing home could not always direct person-

**Table 3.2.   Prevalence of Common Ties Between
Friendship Dyads in The Nursing Home. (N = 110; Sample
B)**

Ties	Percent of Friendship Dyads with Tie Present
Demographic Ties	
Age	70% (77)
Religion	59% (65)
Ethnicity	42% (46)
Prior Occupation/Profession	59% (65)
Preadmission Residence	40% (44)
Family Ties	
Marital Status	58% (64)
Presence or Absence of Children	51% (56)
Nursing Home Ties	
Contemporaneous Tenure	36% (40)
Unit Location	87% (96)
Past Acquaintance	9% (10)

nel to comfort residents whose friends had gone to the hospital; but residents themselves comforted each other. In a nursing home, the designation of "helper" and "helped" blurs because all residents, by definition, require at least minimal help. Residents themselves, however, often helped each other.

Nursing Home Friends

Friendships exist within The Nursing Home, as they exist in countless other nursing homes. Participant observation studies note the existence of friendships among residents. In fact, researchers analyzing "quality of life" within nursing homes have included friendships among their evaluation criteria.[17]

The interesting fact about nursing home friendships is not so much that they exist, but that we don't envision them as we conjure up images of "the nursing home." To some extent, our myopia reflects the notion that a nursing home is preeminently an "institution," and as an institution it so depersonalizes residents that they can no longer function as empathic social beings. We think, in short, that friendships do not happen within the nursing home because conviviality itself is antithetical to institutional, routinized order. So when we look at nursing homes we see only morose, uncommunicative patients who stare at the walls; we overlook the residents who talk to each other.

We also may think that the institutionalized elderly no longer want friends. In the 1960s gerontologists described the "disengagement" of the elderly person who, as functional ability declined, concomitantly withdrew from social life, so that a narrowed social world reflected the individual's own narrowing interests.[18] Retirement, inactive community memberships, and fewer social outings all mark the disengagement of the individual from the larger society. If disengagement theory validly explains the constriction of the social circle of the elderly—and gerontologists[19] have criticized the theory—then the social isolation of the nursing home resident would mark yet one more stage of withdrawal.

Finally, we may overlook the presence of friendships in nursing homes because our calculus of the "needs" of elderly people places such a low emphasis on friendships. We, the nonelderly, think that the elderly need nursing care and nutritious food and family love, but not necessarily friends. Hence, in the nursing home we see only that the nursing home resident is cut off from life within a family, not that the resident may enjoy contact with contemporaries.

Ironically, when we dismiss the importance of friendships for elderly nursing home residents, we in effect equate their social needs with those of infants. We understand that the newborn depends totally upon its family for physical as well as emotional needs. The toddler may sense the existence of "secondary others" beyond the "significant others" who are his family, but he approaches strangers gingerly, even strangers who are the same size and shape as he. Once the child can talk, however, he soon recognizes that very special people exist outside the family circle: friends. Indeed, psychologists have charted the process of "individuation" as the individual family member develops an identity apart from the larger kin unit. In this process of individuation, friendships are critical. The friend, particularly the contemporary friend, becomes a "significant other" important to the personality development of the individual. Typically, adolescents rely even more intensely on peers than on family; and, in post-adolescence, the individual will find a prospective mate from among his/her peers.

Even without the imprimatur of psychologists, however, most people intuitively recognize the need for friends.

As Robert Frost said, "Something there is that doesn't love a wall . . ." We build our walls, if not physical ones, then psychological ones; yet we struggle at the same time to build bonds of intimacy, in spite of the very barriers we erect against that intimacy. A friend may be a relative. Many people enjoy wonderful marriages based on friendship. Parents and their adult children often befriend each other. Years after childhood bickering, siblings may discover that they truly enjoy each other's company. The person without a friend seems bizarre—akin to Camus' Stranger.

Not surprisingly, research on the social supports of the noninstitutionalized elderly has emphasized the importance of friendships. Diverse researchers examining quality of life among the elderly have found that contemporary friends may provide more solace and joy than families.[20] Looking at life within an elderly housing complex, Arlie Hochschild[21] found an "unexpected community" of women who were friends. Although on one hand Hochschild did not find the strong family ties that might seem essential to a full life, she did find strong "sibling" bonds in this collection of women who happened to live in the same building.

Although we recognize the need for friends among children, adolescents, young adults, even among elderly non-institutionalized people, we downplay the need for friends among institutionalized populations. We portray the need for family as paramount for them, much as we would for infants. We see the nursing home as a separation from vital family ties, not as an introduction to a world of possible friends, as it well may be. To return to the title of this book, "Mom" may no longer live among relatives; but in the nursing home she will not be isolated. She will be living among contemporaries some of whom may, in time, become her friends.

Chapter 4

An   Identity

The question remains: Does the nursing home harbor beneath its institutional facade a familial community? The existence of friendships constitutes necessary, but not truly sufficient, evidence. Friendships are important. They testify to the ability of people to form satisfying bonds with those around them; but a community that purports to offer a quasi "home" will at the same time offer some attributes of a family. More specifically, an institution houses inmates·whose primary identity derives from their niches within the institutional world. They are known for what they do, how they behave, or where they live within the institution itself. Their pasts— occupations, friends, family, passions, interests—remain cloaked, irrelevant to their current lives. A family, on the other hand, encompasses individuals with histories. If patients in nursing homes have *de facto* forfeited their pasts, then the nursing home remains far truer to Goffman's asylum than to a family paradigm. In a communal home, those residents will retain the personal histories that they forged throughout their lifetimes.

The forfeit of a personal history is frightening. In the 1960s a BBC television series, "The Prisoner," featured a British foreign intelligence official who suddenly and inexplicably resigned. Because he would not divulge his reasons for doing this, his superiors exiled him to the Village, an idyllic grouping of homes, beaches, and gardens set on an island. Villagers enjoyed a pleasant schedule of bridge, parades, parties, chess games, dances, and concerts , but they could not leave the island. Known by numbers, Village people did not mention past families, jobs, political affiliations, or experiences. "Number 35" played bridge with "Number 27." Only rarely, after a cryptic reference to "the admiral" or a national capital, did the audience glimpse a Villager's past. Repeatedly, the protagonist objected, "I am a person, not a number;" and the sequence of shows detailed the prisoner's ill-plotted schemes to escape the idyllic place where he could only be a number. Life in the Village was pleasant, perhaps pleasanter than in London; yet the prisoner raged against the forfeit of identity.

Nursing homes are hardly so idyllic as the prisoner's island, yet casual onlookers, as well as gerontologists, sociologists, and psychologists, would see the forfeit of identity as a common denominator in both places. The reasons for entering a nursing home vary: some residents are moribund; others live far from potential caregivers; others have outlived caregivers; still others are deranged. Whatever the route, however, the individual becomes a "resident," and that identity overshadows, even eclipses, any prior identity. In nursing homes people are identified by disability, by nursing needs, by room number, perhaps even by physician. Mrs. Smith becomes "the self-care patient on Unit 3," or "the woman with MS," or "one of Dr. Jones' patients." Mr. Morgan becomes the "terminal case in Room 26."

Patients fear this loss of identity, and the fear is justifiable. To the questions, "Who am I?" "What is my essence as a human?" individuals living in the community can cite a range of social roles: mother, spouse, gardener, musician, teacher, nurse, as well as a range of likes and dislikes. Every nursing home resident had a "community" identity that reflected the niche s/he occupied within the noninstitutional world that was home for as many as 80 years. Individuals living in a nursing home may feel they have forfeited that identity to adopt one appropriate to their new world, that they have, in short, traded names for numbers, much like Villagers in the television series.

A complex individual does not instantly become "a resident." For many people the first step in losing their community identity comes before nursing home admission. We construct our identities and our self-images in relationship to a world of others. Friends, spouses, children, siblings, and co-workers all anchor us within the community. When they die, we have lost those valuable anchors who gave our self-conceptions legitimacy. According to Mead's[1] theory of a looking-glass self, people form self-images by seeing themselves through the eyes of others: the images others have are reflected back, in a metaphorical looking glass, to answer for the onlooker, "Who am I?" Without significant others, the individual has no convenient frames of reference. Bishop Barkley debated the phenomenon of a tree falling in a forest. With nobody to hear the crash, does the tree in fact make a noise? So, too, can a person maintain an identity as a social being when all the people integral to that identity have gone?

Indeed, the individual with no significant others has few opportunities for acting out those social roles that comprise an identity. A woman cannot be a spouse, sibling, friend, or parent without others. Many hobbies are solitary activities; but the gardener who has nobody to admire her garden, the cook who has nobody to share her food, even the traveller who has no companion to hear his adventures, have relinquished some of the joy of their avocations. Residents, moreover, have accumulated the memories that define their pasts. To cite Thomas Hood: "I remember, I remember/The house where I was born . . ." Unfortunately, many elderly people have lost the friends and families who shared those memories. Some newly-admitted nursing home residents have no friends or families; indeed, the absence of caregivers may have prompted them to enter a nursing home. Nobody who is now alive knows them. They enter the nursing home with their prior identities compromised, at least partially buried with the people from their past.

For those newly-admitted residents who have both friends and families, nursing home admission marks a physical separation from "significant others." Nursing homes prescribe visiting hours when residents can see the people who have known them, but outside of those hours new residents live among people who do not know them, who have never known them, and may be disinterested in ever knowing anything about them beyond medication needs or room location. Even during visiting hours, moreover, the resident does not fill social roles with friends and families. Relationships—mother and child, brother and sister, grandchild and grandparent—become formalized into visitor and visitee. Small day rooms rarely offer privacy from either fellow residents or omnipresent staff, and visits in patient rooms rarely allow for intimacy if a roommate is present. Stilted conversation must either include the roommate or ignore him/her.

The resident eager to retain a "community" identity will miss the presence of people who had known him or her. The resident will also miss the trappings of that identity. We furnish our homes with reminders and mementoes of our individual histories. Even commonplace furniture will carry memories: the gash from a child's roller skate, the cigarette stain from a party, the light switch that has baffled every handyman. We are comfortable among "familiar" objects; indeed, the word "familiar" has the same Latin root (*familia*) as "family." Objects and people anchor us within a specific niche of the community. We know who we are when we look upon the people and trappings that comprise our small niche. In the nursing home both anchors are gone.

The nursing home substitutes uniform trappings, chosen for sturdiness, efficiency, and ease of manipulation, not aesthetics. Beds, chairs, night tables, bureaus, drapes—all are invariably utilitarian, rarely charming. Nursing homes may hang paintings on walls, but these are usually nondescript, inoffensive, and pedestrian. Some nursing homes provide clothing for residents, but, again, the clothes are chosen for utility and durability. The woman who has lived amidst possessions accumulated during decades of housekeeping may find the spartan nursing home decor especially demoralizing.

The spartan decor, moreover, is uniform. Furniture, room layout, wall hangings—all are similar. To a new resident, Room 38 is indistinguishable from Room 5, and one corridor looks very much like another. Admittedly, a nursing home cannot easily recreate the personal space the person knew within the community; yet nursing homes could be more flexible in enabling residents to demarcate their own private space in their new home.

If people and possessions signal one's community identity, so does one's name. Nursing homes do not, of course, call residents by numbers, but most nursing homes, in a superficial stab at conviviality, drop residents' last names. Mrs. Smith becomes "Mary;" Mr. Jones, "Harry." Over time, long-term residents may *want* staff and fellow residents to use their first names; but using them from the moment the resident enters the nursing home may seem like a subtle put-down to some patients. The first names often become a mnemonic code for staff keen on placing residents within the nursing home schedule: Mary and Harry need physical therapy; George has a G-tube, etc. In nursing homes that serve an array of ethnic populations, a last name suggests the individual's ethnic identity: Mrs. Giordano is probably Italian; Mr. O'Brien, Irish. Without last names, residents have lost audible reminders of their ethnic heritages.

In the television series "The Prisoner," Village prisoners adopted a new identity appropriate to their new life in the Village. Villagers worked as shopkeepers, custodians, lifeguards, cooks, mailmen, physicians. Outside work, villagers were supposed to develop avocations; people painted, gardened, jogged, bicycled, played chess, and organized parties. Thus, the Village strived to let each person develop a new, if limited, identity. Nursing homes separate the individual from a past identity, but, unlike the Village, nursing homes do not foster new identities. For "short-stayers," the reason lies partly in the "sick role." People who are ill are filling a "sick role," to use Parsons'[2] terminology; and the sick role saps the individual's time and energy. According to the requisites of the "sick role," the individual is supposed to concentrate on the prescribed regimen that, ideally, will ameliorate the illness. "Short-stayers" who use the nursing home for convalescence after hospitalization are filling the "sick role." For them, the nursing home offers the trained assistance, medications, and the help with daily tasks that will enable them to "get better." A person filling the sick role will concentrate primarily on getting better. For "short-stayers," nursing home life may mark a loss of community identity, but the loss is perceived as temporary, and residents accept the loss much as they would in a hospital.

"Long-stayers" do not fill the sick role *per se*. The sick role presupposes not only that a patient is ill, but that a patient's compliance with a prescribed regimen will help the patient get better. Although many long-stayers are severely ill and functionally limited, they are not expected to improve. The nursing home is not so much their therapeutic way-station as their actual home. Nursing homes, however, are programmed to fill the needs primarily of people immersed in "the sick role," i.e., people who are concentrating on getting better. Nursing homes not only look like hospitals, but they operate as hospitals. Like hospitals, nursing homes concentrate on the physical and safety needs of residents; recreational and social needs are secondary. Consequently, the nursing home offers few opportunities for residents to do anything other than sit, eat, bathe, pray, and play bingo. Model nursing homes may encourage residents to play musical instruments, write articles, draw, garden, paint, sew, go on outings, or care for a pet; but more plebian nursing homes rarely encourage residents to grow and learn and experience. In most nursing homes individuals—even "long-stayers"—are, primarily, patients. The nursing home in *Limbo,* Carobeth Laird's[3] odyssey, only reluctantly, after much entreating, provided paper and space for her to type the manuscript that recounted that odyssey. Staff neither understood nor cooperated in her desire to develop a new identity through the avocation of writing.

Residents' Histories

The Nursing Home has at any given time approximately 155 residents, each with a long, complex history filled with people, crises, happiness, disasters. The median age of residents is 83. During those many years some residents' lives mirrored soap operas; others, romantic novels. Two residents immigrated in a scenario reminiscent of a spy thriller: Ho Chin W. left China, where he had been politically active, and settled in the United States as a young man. His wife remained in China. When politicians from an opposing party came to power, they took revenge on him. One day he opened a parcel mailed from China to find some of his wife's remains carefully packed. In this country he owned several restaurants, married, raised children, and had grandchildren. Now, at age 88, he lives on a ICF I unit of the nursing home. Another resident, Sylvia A., had been orphaned as a small child when the Turkish forces routed Soviet Armenia. Eventually a nomadic band of Syrians found her and, later, adopted her. At age 85, she still has the characteristic tattoos used by the Syrians to protect her from maurauding Turkish troops.

Other immigrants' histories testify, not to political upheavals, but to the arduous search for prosperity and family, two goals that often did not mesh. Anna G. and Grace P. both left Italy as young girls, settled in this country, worked in textile mills, married, raised families, lost spouses and several children, all the while working at least part-time in the ubiquitous mills. The women lived through two major wars, two relatively minor wars, the Depression, and periods of prosperity that never truly included them in the economic upturns. When women got the vote, Anna and Grace voted for Roosevelt—a rational choice, since their retirement income would mostly consist of the Social Security payments that began with Roosevelt. Perhaps contrary to their dreams as young immigrants, more than 70 years in America did not make them wealthy. They did, however, establish large families, who regularly visit.

In this working class city, few residents held professional jobs; but not everybody worked in textile mills or jewelry factories. Suffering from Alzheimer's disease, Paul V. now sits quacking like a duck as nurses feed him. He used to be a Protestant minister with an advanced degree in English literature and a keen interest in archaeology. Matilda W. listens quietly to the television in her room. A widow with no children, she rarely has visitors. She came to this country as a refugee from Germany. Once here, she found work as a dressmaker, then progressed to fashion designer and theatrical costumer. Her husband, an artist, had painted the wall mural that graces the lobby of the state's oldest fashionable hotel. Several women were registered nurses: one had been chief nurse at a state hospital. They continue to oversee the ministrations of the nursing home's staff from a critical, experienced perspective. Martha J. taught elementary school for over 40 years. Ray G., a local politico who served on local political committees as well as on the city council, had run for mayor. Sven B. had worked as a carpenter. Marjorie C. worked as a maid for a series of wealthy families before becoming a cook in a fashionable resort restaurant. Thomas M. had been a Catholic priest.

Even those women whose lives revolved around domestic chores and responsibilities had often been lead characters in their own family sagas. Women suffered with alcoholic, abusive husbands, raised retarded children who themselves are now institutionalized, mourned the deaths of their children, survived the destitution of the Depression, cared for their own aging parents, divorced, remarried, were widowed. Some married childhood sweethearts and continued to be in love throughout 50-year marriages. Other women never married, but remained close to siblings and parents. The history of each resident is a rich and unique tapestry that s/he brings to the nursing home. The question, of course, is whether anybody knows about this tapestry.

The popular view is that the tapestry is buried prematurely when people enter a nursing home. People live physically, yet their pasts have died. People are known by their disabilities, much like patients in a hospital; yet, where hospital stays last a few weeks, nursing home stays last as long as five years. In a hospital, moreover, patients easily accept an identity delineated by name tags and code words. In an institution that purportedly offers a home, individuals demur at the identification codes and forms. Residents who have already suffered innumerable losses, from spouse to home to functional ability, must face a new loss: the loss of self; and that loss may be more frightening and more final than previous losses.

The Search

At The Nursing Home, the search for patient identities began with staff, who were asked what they knew about their patients' past lives. Each staff member was asked to talk about residents whom s/he had worked with for at least eight weeks. Staff on interim or short-term assignments might reasonably know little about residents and were not questioned, but staff who had worked regularly with residents would have had occasion to talk to them, to meet family members, and to read patient charts.

Essentially, staff have three sources of information about patients' pasts. First, from those patients who can communicate. Confused, aphasic, or hearing-impaired residents may be unable to tell staff who they are, what they liked, where they had lived, and what they had done in their lives. Residents who are not so impaired, however, may find staff too occupied doing "bed and body" work to listen. "Psychosocial support" is not considered essential to nursing home job descriptions. In fact, one study[4] charted improvements in patient functioning when selected staff deliberately tried to chat with residents. Such chatter was considered extraneous—it was the "experiment" variable in the controlled study. Another researcher[5] found housekeepers more inclined to talk to residents than the clinical nursing staff assigned to those residents.

The second source of information comes from residents' families. Over time, families become part of the social ambiance of the nursing home. Staff and family members come to know each other, and, ideally, will talk to each other, if not formally in designated conferences, then informally during visits.

The third source of information is the psychosocial history that the social worker compiles at admission. At The Nursing Home, the social worker interviews each newly-admitted resident. If the resident cannot offer a cogent personal history, the social worker will obtain a past history from relatives and friends. The psychosocial history, usually two to three pages long, traces the life of the resident from birth (place, parents' occupation, number of siblings) to schooling to marriage to the workforce to the varied changes in family status (death of siblings, divorce, abuse, children's delinquencies or triumphs). The psychosocial history includes activities the resident enjoyed, special interests s/he had, and interesting experiences the resident or the family member may remember. For some residents the psychosocial history is short. Residents who have trans-

ferred from other nursing homes, who have no close relatives, and who are unable to understand the social worker's
questions will have only a brief notation under "history"—a
notation gleaned from past notes of hospital social workers,
welfare case worker records, and other nursing home social
workers. Alex S. has only a four-line psychosocial history.
He transferred to this nursing home from a state institution, where he had lived for years, and which had misplaced
the records that would offer clues to his birthplace, parents,
age at institutionalization, or reason for institutionalization.
A chance comment from a state social worker suggested
that he may be of Russian extraction; but since he cannot
speak, he can neither corroborate nor deny that one inkling
of a non-institutional history.

The instrument used to interview staff about their
knowledge of their patients' histories consisted of the simple open-ended question, "Please tell me anything you
know about the past life of (patient's name)." Fifty-three
full-time staff members (4 housekeepers, 38 aides/order-
lies, 4 nursing aide coordinators, 5 charge nurses, and 2
head nurses) who had worked at the nursing home at least
four months were interviewed. They gave their assessments
of 130 residents (Sample A) who had lived at the home at
least five months (the director of nurses was excluded).
Staff members were asked only about residents whom
they had worked with directly for at least eight weeks,
even though many on the staff were familiar with other
long-term residents.

The "Historical I"

The search for friendships yielded evidence that nursing
homes may not be so grim as the popular literature
suggests. The search for historical identity was not so re-

warding. Of 130 residents, seven truly had forfeited their pasts. Not one staff member knew anything about them—neither their former occupation, their community involvement, their past family experiences, nor their adventures in life.

Each resident was given a "staff knowledge" score which indicated the percentage of staff workers familiar with the resident who knew some detail of his or her past life. A score of 100% meant that all staff who had worked with a patient knew something about that resident's "historical I." A score of 50% meant that half the staff workers knew some detail. In a family, all members know each other's pasts since they share many of the same frames of reference, survived many of the same experiences, knew the same people. Family members may not necessarily like each other: they may even loathe one another; but even in the most disturbed, incommunicative families, members know each other's histories. Within an archetypic institution, however, people may know nothing about each other's pasts. Much like the characters in the Village, residents are known by their niche within the institution, not the niche they filled in the community.

At this nursing home the median "staff knowledge" score was 22%; the mean, 24%, with a 15% standard deviation. Not one resident had a score of 100%. Even Ho Chin W., the political refugee from China, had at least one staff member who was regularly involved with his care but knew nothing of his past life. For most residents, in short, the "historical I" remained partially hidden. Staff knew room locations of residents, their functional ability, their friends within the nursing home, their particular peeves. Staff also sensed residents' moods, and most staff could describe specific residents' personalities as pleasant, kind, spiteful, good-humored, short-tempered, maternal, and so forth. Many members of the staff, however, did not know whether the resident had worked in a textile mill, had been a teacher, had loved baseball, had travelled widely, had belonged to the Elks, or, as was the case of several residents, had entered this country as a political refugee.

People, Not Numbers

The gloomy finding is that a substantial number of residents did lose their past identities, becoming "the case in Room 132."

Not all residents, however, lost their identities; and the extent to which a resident became a "case" varied. Only 7 of 130 residents were, from a staff perspective, complete enigmas; the remaining 123 residents had at least one staff worker at least nominally familiar with one detail from their past lives.

The search for a familial community within a nursing home seems ill-fated; but sociological tools may prove more enlightening than the simple tabulation of lost identities. The question becomes, not *how many* people have become "cases," but *which* people are most likely to be cases in a nursing home?

To answer that question, a regression equation was constructed. The dependent variable was each resident's "staff knowledge" score. The independent variables included possible factors important in predicting that score, specifically:

Community Ties. Do people with strong ties to the community succeed in retaining their community identity once they live in a nursing home?

Five variables suggested the strength of community ties:

1. *Presence of relatives on staff.* At this nursing home

five residents had relatives on staff. Do such residents retain more of their "historical I" than other residents?

2. *Presence of relatives among the residents.* Many nursing homes have brother and sister combinations, husband and wife duos, and, occasionally, a parent and child. Nineteen residents at The Nursing Home were related. Do staff become more familiar with the pasts of the residents who already have family living in the nursing home?

3. *Frequency of visits.* A scale was developed for each resident. Floor nurses were asked to rate the frequency of visits from the following categories: spouse, children, siblings, extended family members, friends. Visits were rated as Frequent (once a week or more), Regular (once a month yet less than once a week), Occasional (less than once a month), Rarely/Never. A summary index was constructed. Do residents with many visits retain their identities more effectively than less-visited residents?

4. *Presence of living relatives: spouse, children, siblings.* Most relatives of these residents lived within ten miles of The Nursing Home. Are people with living relatives better able to convey a coherent sense of their community identity than people who have no living "significant others"?

5. *Community residence.* Forty-seven percent of the residents came to The Nursing Home, not from their own or a child's home, but from a different nursing home. Are these nursing home veterans at a disadvantage compared to their counterparts who entered this nursing home directly from the community?

Other variables considered included:

Demographic characteristics; specifically:
Age
Sex
Prior occupation (homemaker, unskilled/factory;
    retail/skilled, professional, etc.)

Nursing home data:
Tenure in this nursing home. Do people lose their
    identity the longer they live in a nursing home?
Mental lucidity. The social worker made this determ-
    ination. Residents were rated: lucid all the time,
    sometimes, rarely. This was not an assessment
    of cognitive abilities, but simply an assessment
    of the individual's grasp of who and where s/he
    was, who visitors were, what job s/he had held,
    and so on. The assumption was that individuals
    unable to communicate a coherent sense of their
    "historical I" would be more likely to forfeit their
    past identities than more cogent residents.

A Computer Response

To the question, "What patients are more likely to retain
their identities?" the computer pointed to three major influences: the frequency of visits (beta = .23), the absence
of a living spouse (beta = .23), and having had a skilled
or professional occupation (beta = .36). Table 4.1 summarizes the results of the regression equation.

From the standpoint of resident identity, visits serve
a critical function: they establish an image of the resident
in staff eyes. Through visiting relatives, staff learn about
the resident, giving the resident who has many visits an
advantage over the more isolated resident. If "Mom" wor-

ries that upon entrance to a nursing home she will cease
to be a person in the eyes of staff and will exist simply as
a medical case, family members can reassure her that so
long as relatives visit, staff will in all probability not see
her as just another case. The staff's first image of a resident
is of a sick individual who needs specific medications, a

**Table 4.1   Regression Analysis, Considering Knowledge
about Residents by Staff as the Dependent Variable and
Resident Characteristics as the Independent Variables. (N
= 130; Sample A)**

Resident Characteristics	Knowledge of Residents Beta
Community Ties	
Relatives on Staff	.15**
Relatives as Residents	.14
Frequency of Visits	.23**
No Living Spouse	.23**
No Living Child	.12
No Living Sibling	-.05
Admitted from Community	.13
Demographic Data	
Age	-.08
Male	.15*
Skilled or Professional Occupation	.36**
Nursing Home Data	
Tenure (months) in The Nursing Home	.04
Lucidity	-.15*

$$R^2 = -.30*$$

levels of significance:
    **$p < .001$
     *$p < .05$

specific diet, a specific therapeutic regimen, and who suffers from specific medical ailments. Visits from family can superimpose historical details on that primary image, so that the residents and staff recognize the patient as a complex person with some semblance of a past. In *Limbo*, Carobeth Laird describes the frightening loss of identity she felt when she was transferred from a nursing home near friends to one far from friends. Her family, moreover, had died or was estranged. Carobeth Laird suffered the separation from her "historical self" that only relatives/friends could help her sustain in a nursing home. Her fellow residents who had frequent visits from family members probably did not suffer the same separation.

Another key to retaining a historical self-image is the resident's prior occupation. According to the data, residents with skilled and professional occupations were more likely to retain their "historical I." Perhaps such residents were fond of reminiscing about past work experiences. During their work careers, they may have made more stimulating friends, developed more interests in the world outside their families, and travelled more. Indeed, one staff member speculated on her lack of knowledge about several patients: "I think their lives were just so awful they don't want to remember them."

A surprising finding was that residents with no living spouses had higher staff knowledge scores (beta = .23) than those with living spouses. Widows and spinsters, in short, were better known among staff than were married women.

The regression equation also pointed to the importance of relatives on the staff. Not surprisingly, staff knew more about the residents who were related to people on the staff. The beta (.15), however, though statistically significant at .001, is weaker than the betas of some other independent variables.

Not all statistically significant variables are necessarily valid predictors of resident identity. In a multiple regression equation the sociologist seeks to distinguish the *comparative* predictive value of different independent variables upon a dependent variable—to cull strong relationships from the mass of data. For a useful model of social interaction, the sociologist looks for variables with high betas (at least above .20 and statistically significant at .001). The computer may point to "weak" relationships that may or may not be important in predicting interaction, but whose importance would require further investigation. In this computer-generated model of staff knowledge, the computer isolated two such "weak" variables that may be simply statistical anomalies of the manipulation of data. In other words, they may have no relationship with the dependent variable. First, the regression equation suggests that staff members knew more about the pasts of male residents than of female. The finding is plausible, but since the beta (.15) is low and significant only at the .05 level, no conclusion is possible.

Second, mental lucidity showed an inverse relationship (beta = -.15): the more confused the resident, the more staff members were likely to know something about him/her. This finding is the opposite of what might have been expected since confused residents are unable to communicate a cogent sense of their own pasts to staff and, hence, would seem likely to become nursing home "cases." This startling finding, however, may very well signify the lack of a predictive relationship between the two variables, lucidity and staff knowledge. The value of the beta is low, as is its statistical significance level ($p < .05$). Kadishin,[6] a sociologist, has suggested that researchers establish a *Journal of Nonsignificant Findings* for findings whose lack of significance is surprising. The unimportance, at least statistically, of resident confusion, belongs in such a journal.

Confused residents did not inevitably become "cases."

Nor were nursing home "veterans" more likely to forfeit their pasts. We may think that people lose their identities as they travel from nursing home to nursing home in a kind of institutional nomadism, but the variable, "Admitted from the Community" (beta = .13) shows no statistically significant impact on staff knowledge. People who came to The Nursing Home from a different nursing home, as opposed to directly from the community, were not necessarily "cases" so long as they had family members who visited.

A Staff Link

The computer was also asked whether some staff members were more likely than others to learn about their residents. The typical staff worker at The Nursing Home is a 30-year-old Catholic female aide who has worked at The Nursing Home almost two years and is more likely than not to have living parents and no children. Eighty-five percent of staff interviewed have living mothers; 60% have living fathers. Like the patients, a majority (74%) of staff are Catholic. Again, a multiple regression equation was constructed, with staff knowledge about their patients' pasts the dependent variable and staff characteristics the independent variables. Each staff member had a score: the proportion of his/her residents about whom s/he knew some historical detail. A score of 100% meant that a staff worker knew some detail about all his/her charges; a score of 50% meant that the staff workers knew about the pasts of half his/her charges; a score of 0%, that the staff member knew nothing about the pasts of any residents whom s/he had cared for throughout at least eight weeks.

Independent variables included staff characteristics; specifically, job status, age, sex, tenure at The Nursing Home, and presence of living relatives. Table 4.2 summarizes the results.

The computer pointed to higher-status employees as the most knowledgeable. Charge nurses and registered nurses were more likely to know about their residents' pasts than aides, orderlies, or housekeepers. Although the latter may spend more time chatting with residents, the more credentialled staff may be more likely to read the psychosocial histories included in the social work history portion of patient charts. Also, the computer pointed to childless staff (beta = .33) and staff with no living fathers

---

Table 4.2.   Regression Analysis, Considering Staff Knowledge of Residents' Pasts as the Dependent Variable and Staff Characteristics as the Independent Variables. (N = 53; Sample A)

Staff Characteristics	Knowledge of Residents' Pasts beta
Higher Job Status	.30**
No Living Children	.33*
No Living Father	.22*
Time Employed	.19
Living Spouse	.17
No Living Mother	.14
Age	-.12

$$R^2 = .32$$

levels of significance:
    ** p .001
     * p .05

(beta = .22) as the most knowledgeable; but the level of significance was low.

A Home of Individuals

Hospitals house patients. Nursing homes house residents. If those residents come to the nursing home firmly rooted in their communities, with a strong self-image formed during an interesting work life, they may not suffer that loss of past identity that accompanies "institutionalization."

Nursing home residents may remain individuals, not cases. The evidence from The Nursing Home suggests on one hand that many residents have in fact forfeited much of their historical identities; but, on the other hand, that the forfeit is not inevitable, but depends to some extent on the support of family, the prior occupation of the resident, and the staff practice of reading the intake psychosocial histories. The literature on institutionalization bemoans the loss of historical self as individuals become inmates. In this nursing home, however, some residents—admittedly not enough—did retain the vestiges of a noninstitutional identity in the eyes of staff.

Chapter 5

The Hired Custodians

"It is not that we are afraid to die. It is just that we want someone who cares near us when it happens."—Letter to the Editor, Providence Journal, December 12, 1985.

So wrote an elderly man who echoed a common fear: the fear of dying emotionally alone. To use sociological jargon, people in the community supposedly live amongst "significant others." In a nursing home people live surrounded by hired custodians, "secondary others," who may neither know them nor care for them. If isolation is measured only by the lack of companions, the nursing home resident will not die alone since s/he is surrounded by a bevy of uniformed staff, fellow residents, and visitors; but s/he may die emotionally alone.

In Search of Caring

The literature on nursing homes portrays different archetypical staff members. There is The Sadist, like Nurse Ratchet in *One Flew Over The Cuckoo's Nest*.[1] This worker steals from patients, ignores their desire for privacy, uses their phones, hits them, and threatens them with reprisals if they complain to family or administrators.[2] Increasingly timid and diffident, residents faced with The Sadist escape her abusive ministrations only by going to the hospital or by dying. Then there is The Incompetent, who cannot perform the tasks demanded of her.[3] Under her care patients are more likely to suffer falls, miss medications, have serious bouts of pneumonia go unrecognized, and so on. Unlike The Sadist, The Incompetent may be fond of patients, but her incompetence renders her a menace to their well-being. The Automaton, the third type, looks upon her patients with detachment.[4] She neither likes nor dislikes them, but views them dispassionately, as inert bodies. She performs her routine conscientiously. Although she may appreciate cooperative residents and regret the uncooperative ones, she feels no emotional response to them. Yet the need for love and affection does not diminish as people age. Residents for whom the nursing home is a labor-intensive incubator will grow withdrawn and will see themselves as physical shells for souls that have already died.

Finally, we have The Mother. She infantilizes residents,[5] treating them like "cute," "loveable," "adorable" dolls who, not surprisingly, soon think of themselves as children, unable to make decisions or control their lives. When the "looking glass self" reflects back an incompetent child, a resident may understandably behave like one. This surrogate mother is often a meticulous housekeeper who performs the "bed and body" work on residents with such fervor that they lose the ability to button clothes, feed themselves, or walk unassisted. The more zealously staff members perform duties for residents, the more likely that those residents will cease trying—a loss of functional ability that the literature dubs "induced dependence."[6]

The stereotype of The Mother deserves scrutiny. The literature criticizes aides who infantilize residents by thinking of them as adorable children; and a mother-child model of interaction clearly seems inappropriate for a 25-year-old aide and an 86-year-old widow. Nevertheless, critics do not strongly put forth a "preferred" model of interaction. A formal client-provider interchange seems equally inappropriate, especially when the nursing home staff will be a surrogate family, at least in terms of time spent together, for the resident's last years. And the maternal aide at least manifests an emotional response to her patients. Many of the aides who speak so fondly of their patients also speak of them as quasi-children—not an irrational response given the dependence of the elderly person on the aide for help with the most basic tasks of daily living. While it is easy to criticize such a maternal stance, the stance bespeaks genuine affection; and in a facility where people fear dying "emotionally alone," that affection deserves recognition.

As for induced dependence, while it may be fashionable to criticize aides who overzealously button shirts, feed meals, and wheel chairs, it is unfair to do so. The line between promoting independence and overlooking residents' needs for help blurs. Contemporary medicine is embued with an activist enthusiasm for restoring health, curing illness, and overcoming disability. Such enthusiasm may be misplaced in nursing homes. The vast majority of residents enter nursing homes with no discharge planned. They enter, moreover, at least partly because they cannot function in the community. In short, they need help. To criticize aides for helping "too much" asks from staff an uncanny ability to demarcate the point where helping is harmful. An aide who is faulted for feeding a resident (the sin of inducing dependence) may just as easily be faulted for not feeding a resident (the

sin of neglecting or even abusing). Similarly, the truism
that aides should "encourage" residents to do as much
as possible does not offer clear guidelines as to how
much, how long, and with what consequences. Although
the aide should offer encouragement, no guidelines
specify how much encouragement. After one suggestion
that the resident feed himself, should the staff member
then offer to feed the resident? After three suggestions?
Should the staff member let the resident miss a meal
before lifting a spoon? Two meals? Staff who know residents may sense their capabilities. Indeed, The Nursing
Home's staff believed that some of the most disliked
residents did not do as much as they were able; but, from
the stance of a sociological investigation of a nursing
home, the charge of induced dependence is difficult to
define or measure.

That there are disparate "types" of aides is not surprising because the perception of the role of staff in a
nursing home is not clear. The hospital model holds staff
responsible primarily for specific instrumental tasks.
Much like hospital staff, nursing home staff must compe-
tently and conscientiously perform "bed and body work"
on residents, monitor medications, and carry out prescribed therapeutic regimens. Residents for their part
may expect no more from staff. In a long-term facility,
however, the strict hospital model seems inadequate, if
only because staff will be in contact with residents for
the rest of their lives—far more in terms of hours per
week than families.

Hovering behind all these images is the demographic profile of the nursing home worker as a mini-
mally-paid, minimally-trained, minimally-credentialled
female shouldered with an almost Herculean daily work
regimen of tasks and responsibilities. She often chooses

the nursing home because she lacks sufficient credentials or experience for a more lucrative hospital job.

The search for a familial community within The Nursing Home spurred a sociological investigation of two prevalent myths: first, the notion of automaton-like residents staring vacantly ahead, not relating to one another, unable to form meaningful relationships; and, second, the notion that upon entering a nursing home residents abandon their past identities, in a kind of institutionalization rite that transforms individuals into "cases." The pervasive stereotypes of abusive/unfeeling/inept/harmful staff deserve similar sociological probing.

Staff affect—or the absence thereof—toward residents is not self-evident to casual visitors, who see only the bustle of staff intent on completing specifically delineated tasks. Do staff, like Nurse Ratchet, despise residents? Do staff consider their residents "adorable?" Or do staff members, construing their jobs as instrumental tasks to be performed efficiently on inert bodies, find the question of emotional attachment irrelevant?

Anecdotes are the first key to staff feelings. And The Nursing Home yields a plethora of anecdotes that suggest how warmly staff feel towards their charges. Karen X., a 23-year-old unmarried nurse's aide on an intermediate level unit, took Mr. and Mrs. S. home to her family for Thanksgiving dinner when Karen learned that the S. children would not be visiting their parents on Thanksgiving. Mrs. S. is so confused that staff doubt that she recognizes her own family, but Karen believes that Mrs. S. recognizes her. Mr. S. is incontinent. Susan Y., another aide, occasionally takes Bessie M. home for Sunday dinner. Susan lives with her machinist husband and several small children in a house near the nursing home. As a special treat, Anne Z., a nurse's aide, occasionally takes Jean W. to a nearby movie. Lucille L. is a middle-aged alcoholic, comatose for over a year, presumably because she combined drugs and alcohol in a particularly toxic way. At first her husband used to visit and talk to her. After several months her husband and his girlfriend began to visit less frequently. When they stopped visiting, Mildred A., a middle-aged aide, began a routine of daily five-minute chatty monologues at Lucille's bedside. One aide gave Sarah B. a parakeet for a present. Often staff members grieve when a resident dies. These anecdotes, while not frequent, are not rare. Indeed, participant observation studies of nursing homes have remarked on the gentleness and caring of some staff members.

Nursing notes enhance the anecdotal evidence. When Alex M., a former resident of a state mental institution, had to go to the hospital, the notes report staff pleasure when he returned "home to us." Staff reportedly "enjoy Hannah J.'s wonderful sense of humor." In nursing records staff voice indignation at children they perceive as insufficiently concerned about their resident parents.

Ancedotal evidence, however, yields a skewed portrait of nursing staff. Like Pollyanna, staff and administrators remember the most cheerful anecdotes, the kindest nurses, the friendliest relationships. To give a more realistic, and truer, portrait of staff feelings, information must embrace a wider sample of staff and residents. In this case, 53 full-time clinical and housekeeping staff members who had worked at The Nursing Home at least four months were interviewed concerning residents who had been at the home at least five months. Each worker was asked, simply, "How would you feel if patient X transferred to another facility?" (Nursing home transfers occur routinely; in fact, every time a resident enters the hospital, s/he enters a nursing home lottery where a bed in a specific nursing home may or may not be available.) Staff were asked to decide: 1) Would you be pleased at the transfer? 2) Would you have no strong reaction one way or the other? 3) Would you miss the resident? Each resident was given three scores: 1, the "negative affect score"—the percent of staff eager for the resident to leave the nursing home; 2, the "object affect" score—the percent of staff who felt indifferently towards the resident; and 3, the "positive affect" score—the percent of staff who would truly miss the resident. Each staff member was interviewed individually, in a closed session; and, aware that nobody would be identified by name, they were encouraged to respond honestly.

The sample of patients studied included only the 130 people who had lived at The Nursing Home for at least 5 months (Sample A)—the "long-stayers." Presumably staff might not develop strong feelings for new residents. Nor would staff feel strongly towards the residents who die shortly after admission. For "long-stayers," however, the formation of emotional bonds among staff and residents seems natural.

The results of the survey suggest that staff have positive feelings toward residents. (See Table 5.1.)

**Table 5.1.   Affect Scores Received by Patients.
(N = 130; Sample A)**

	Mean	Median	Standard Deviation
Negative Affect Score	10%	6%	13%
Object Affect Score	33%	32%	16%
Positive Affect Score	57%	59%	15%

Negative affect scores. The negative affect scores isolate residents whom staff actively dislike. The scores show the proportion of staff who commonly work with that resident who want him/her to transfer elsewhere. A 50% score for

a patient would mean that 50% of the staff involved in
that patient's care would be pleased at his/her transfer. As
Table 5.1 shows, few patients were so actively and generally
disliked. The mean negative affect score was 10%; the median, 6%—a marked contrast to the mean positive affect
score (57%). In short, an average resident would find that
over half the staff who had worked with the resident was
fond of him/her. Although staff did not react uniformly
to all patients, a high negative correlation between positive
and negative affect (-.71) and between positive and object
affect (-.87) exists. (See Table 5.2 for correlation matrix.)
Fifty residents (36% of the sample) had no staff member
who wanted him/her to transfer. Only six residents had
negative affect scores above 35%, meaning that more than
a third of the staff working with these patients wanted
them transferred. A resident who fears spending a life
among people who loathe him/her can probably relax. At
this nursing home, at least, the staff's "negative affect" towards patients was very low.

**Table 5.2.   Correlation Matrix of Staff Affect
Scores (N = 130; Sample A)**

	Positive Affect	Object Affect	Negative Affect
Positive Affect	—	-.87	-.71
Object Affect		—	.26
Negative Affect			—

Object affect scores. The second question ("Would you
have no strong reaction one way or the other if the patient
were to transfer?") tried to tap the phenomenon of institu-

tional affect, where staff, according to Goffman, view residents with detached objectivity. Staff may behave conscientiously towards residents, and may enjoy their jobs, but they develop no strong emotional bonds with residents. Many prospective nursing home residents and their families have visited friends and relatives already living in nursing homes. These visitors may recognize that The Sadist is a myth, but they fear The Automaton who, as the letter writer quoted at the beginning of this chapter seemed to imply, works with the resident but cares nothing about him or her.

The object affect scores signify the proportion of staff who are so detached from the resident that a transfer would neither please nor displease them. Within a classic institution, inmates are objects; and, while staff are supposed to treat inmates fairly, skillfully, and "professionally," the very norm of professional behavior implies an emotional detachment. Emotional detachment is not necessarily evil. The counterpart to such a norm is personal favoritism toward clients. A physician, for instance, should not love some patients and abhor others, but should sublimate emotional reactions, treating all patients courteously and responsively, yet uniformly. Similarly, hospital nursing staff are not faulted for a detached stance, assuming their behavior is courteous.

A nursing home, however, is not a hospital; and while hospital stays might average less than two weeks, nursing home stays may average over a year. At The Nursing Home the median stay was 29 months. Some residents had lived there over four years. The norm of professional detachment, appropriate for hospital nursing staff, may not be appropriate or desirable in a long-term care facility, where many patients need custodial care rather than skilled nursing services. And if the facility purports to offer some sort of familial community to its residents, emotional detachment mocks that purported goal.

In this nursing home most staff did not see residents with detached objectivity. The mean object affect score was 33%; the median, 32%.

Positive affect scores. If a classic "institution" would be expected to show a preponderance of staff who felt detached from its inmates, then a classic "familial community" would be expected to show a preponderance who felt positive affect toward residents. In a truly familial community people should feel emotional reactions towards one another—not simply residents toward fellow residents, but staff toward residents. As the positive affect scores suggest, the majority of staff were fond of the majority of residents. If an average resident transferred, more than half of the staff would miss him/her.

The Loved Resident

The literature yields no clear portrait of nursing home residents. Demographically, we know that nursing home residents are likely to be old: 20% of people aged 85 or older live in nursing homes.[7] We know also that these people usually suffer from a combination of chronic debilitating illnesses: new residents' intake diagnoses often present a medical menu of disabilities. We know dementia and confusion are present in a substantial number of these complex diagnostic assessments. We know too that nursing homes house more women than men, and more white women than black women, even considering population proportions. Comparing elderly people living in the community and elderly people living in nursing homes, we know that the "coping ability" (admittedly an ability which is impossible to define quantitatively or definitively) of patient families is an important distinguishing characteristic, more important than the functional ability of the patient.[8] We do not know, however, which people are more likely to find emotional satisfaction in the nursing home, or why some residents find caring people in the nursing home while others live there emotionally isolated.

To construct a clearer portrait of the "loved" resident, the computer was enlisted as the electronic seer. Each resident was given a total affect score: for each staff worker involved with a resident who reported that s/he would miss the resident if he or she transferred to another nursing home, the resident received a +1 score. The sum of the +1 scores represented the total number of workers who reported some positive feeling for that resident. For each staff worker who reported no strong feeling, the resident received no points. And for each staff worker who reported that s/he would be pleased were the resident to transfer, the resident received a −1 score. In short, a summary index was constructed by adding positive scores to negative scores. The total was divided by the number of staff involved with that particular resident. The resulting number signified an "affect scale" for each resident. The highest score on the scale was +1. A resident with a +1 score would be liked by all staff involved in his/her care. The lowest score was −1. Such a resident would be universally disliked.

Scale of Affect: _____

$$-1 \qquad\qquad 0 \qquad\qquad +1$$
negative affect   object affect   positive affect

To determine resident characteristics that influenced staff affect, a multiple regression equation was constructed. Resident affect scores were the dependent variable. Independent variables included the resident's age, sex, prior occupation, pre-admission residence (from the community or from another nursing home), lucidity, tenure within this nursing home, the frequency of visits, the existence of living family, and the presence of relatives either among staff or residents. The list of independent variables replicated the list of independent variables used in the multiple regression equation that considered staff knowledge of patients' past histories (Table 4.1) as the dependent variable—with one exception. In this equation of affect, staff

Table 5.3.   Regression Analysis, Considering Staff Affect Scores as the Dependent Variable and Resident Characteristics as the Independent Variables. (N = 130; Sample A)

Resident Characteristics	Staff Affect Toward Residents Beta
Staff Knowledge about Resident	.24*
Patient Lucidity	.21*
Frequency of Visits	.18
No Relatives on Staff	.14
No Relatives as Residents	.12
Age	-.10
Admitted from Other Nursing Home	.07
No Living Child	.07
No Living Spouse	.06
Tenure (months) in The Nursing Home	-.04
Unskilled Prior Occupation	.03
Male	.02
No Living Sibling	.02

$$R^2 = .17$$

level of significance
   * p .001

knowledge was itself considered an independent variable. In short, the proportion of staff who were knowledgeable about a given resident's past history was included as a plausible variable that might influence staff affect.

The results of the multiple regression equation (Table 5.3) suggest a portrait of the loved resident. The strongest betas were staff knowledge (.24) and resident lucidity (.21).

In Figure 5.1 the regression coefficients for the equation where knowledge of residents' pasts was the dependent variable (described in Chapter 4) and where affect was the independent variable have been used to construct a path model of positive staff affect. The model shows variables both directly and indirectly important in predicting staff affect scores. The loved resident is, generally, a resident who has retained a vestige of identity. Staff knowledge was the greatest predictor of positive staff affect; in other words, staff felt most positively toward residents whom they knew as individuals with pasts, not simply cases.

A key predictor of staff knowledge was the frequency of visits, which in turn depended upon the existence of living family members. Most family members lived within a ten-mile radius of The Nursing Home. The fear that an individual will lose his/her identity in a nursing home and will die emotionally alone, surrounded by an aloof staff, is not groundless, but the statistical evidence from this nursing home suggests that people with strong family supports are less likely to live out their lives as "cases" among staff automatons.

Staff also felt positively toward lucid residents. Participant observation studies of nursing homes have documented the unpopularity of disoriented, confused, deranged residents among fellow residents. Indeed, lucid residents may grow depressed living beside deranged residents. Given the unpopularity of confused residents among their lucid peers, the finding that confused resi-

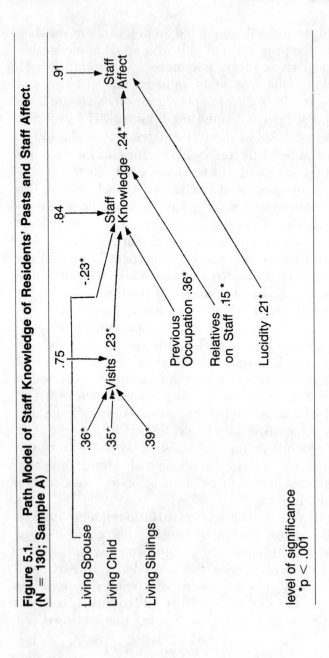

**Figure 5.1. Path Model of Staff Knowledge of Residents' Pasts and Staff Affect.
(N = 130; Sample A)**

Living Spouse

Living Child

Living Siblings

.36*

.35†

.39*

Visits .23*

.75

-.23*

.84

Staff
Knowledge

.91

Staff
Affect

Previous
Occupation .36*

Relatives
on Staff .15 *

Lucidity .21*

Knowledge .24*

level of significance
*p < .001

dents are less popular among staff, while disconcerting, is not surprising.

Tenure in the nursing home showed no impact upon staff affect. Loved residents were not loved because over time staff grew fond of them.

Just as data on staff were analyzed to predict whether some staff members would be more likely than others to learn patient histories (Chapter 4), so too staff data were analyzed to note whether some staff showed more affect towards residents than other staff—in short, whether variations in staff affect depended upon staff characteristics as well as resident characteristics.

In this instance the computer responded, "no." No staff characteristic proved a significant predictor of staff affect. Neither job status, time employed, age, the presence of living relatives, or staff knowledge influenced staff affect.

Disliked Patients

Genuine staff antipathy towards residents existed. Although the number of disliked residents was small at The Nursing Home (the median score on negative staff affect was 6%), several residents scored above 50% on the index; that is, over half of the staff working with those residents wanted them to transfer to another nursing home. These are the residents discussed informally on breaks, when staff complain among themselves. Although staff antipathy may not necessarily affect staff attentiveness, meticulousness, or judgment, antipathy remains a problem—both for the disliked residents, whose quality of life is diminished when caregivers feel strong antipathy, as well as for staff themselves. A key reward of working in a nursing home comes not from salary or fringe benefits, but from the

satisfaction of helping residents.[9] When caregivers dislike
the people they care for, staff morale plummets.

Theoretically the explanation for staff antipathy to
particular residents should lie either with the resident, with
the staff member, or with their interaction.

"Resident-centered" hypotheses center on resident
characteristics that trigger staff dislike. Outside the walls
of the nursing home, staff and residents freely choose their
companions, but the closed nature of the home mandates
continued contact, even for incompatible people. Disliked
residents may be belligerent, mean, irascible, or argumen-
tative. Such residents may plausibly arouse staff antipathy.
Indeed, some residents' disagreeable personalities prompted their families to seek custodial care. Differences in
personality remain a fact. Even children differ in "loveable-
ness" and "cuddliness."

The staff member's personality is also a factor. Just
as residents can be irascible, mean, and belligerent, so too
can staff. Nursing homes where most staff members actively dislike their residents may have a preponderance of
misanthropic staff.

Racial and class differences between staff and residents may explain antipathy. If either residents or staff
regard the other as inferior, that intolerance can disinte-
grate into dislike.[10]

Finally, the interaction between residents and staff may
lead to antipathy. Within a nursing home both the staff
and the residents fill specific roles, with duties and obligations. Staff must enforce the nursing home routine; and
residents who dislike the fact of institutionalization, the
omnipresent companions, the monotonous routines, even
the food, may see staff attentions as yet another intrusion
on their privacy as well as another reminder of their diminished autonomy. Indeed, participation observation
studies have highlighted the frustration that individuals

feel on entering a nursing home—a frustration that residents may translate into anger or bitterness. These residents may complain, resist, yell, remain indifferent to the most attentive staff. Over time, a worker can understandably resent such a resident.

Staff may dislike residents who do not accept their role of patient. The resident who refuses medications, disregards housekeeping schedules, flaunts visiting rules, and balks at prescribed activities like physical therapy will be hindering staff efficiency and, perhaps, work evaluations.

To develop a portrait of the disliked resident, the six residents—all women—with negative affect scores above 35% were identified. One resident scored 75% on negative affect: three-quarters of the staff involved with her care wanted her to transfer. In open-ended interviews, three nursing home staff members—the director of nurses, the social worker, and a long-time charge nurse—speculated on each resident's marked unpopularity. Only the charge nurse had responded to the initial interview on staff knowledge and staff affect. Table 5.4 summarizes content analysis of their responses.

These unpopular residents frustrated staff efforts at caregiving. They were unappreciative, ungrateful, belligerent, and hampered staff desires to feel useful. The ungrateful and complaining family of one resident aggravated staff reaction to the resident herself. These six were not the most difficult to care for, nor the most disagreeable, but they were the least appreciative.[11] Respondents felt that staff tolerated belligerence, ill humor, and heavy caregiving demands when residents occasionally said thank you or a kind word. Understandably, many residents are too depressed to focus on the feelings of staff aides; and, in these instances, respondents emphasized the importance of family-staff relationships. An understanding family with an occasional kind word for an aide will make that aide

Table 5.4. **Content Analysis of Key Staff Questionnaires.**
(Sample A)

	Residents					
	A	B	C	D	E	F
Combative Behavior (bites/hits)	1	3				4
Complains	1				2	
Demands Attention	3		2		3	
Whines		1				
Has "No Personality"		1				
Has Physical Deformity			1			
Is Hysterical at Rapid Debilitation				2	1	
Staff Feel Impotent to Help or Please	3	3	3	2	2	
Is Ungrateful	2	2	2		2	
Has Complaining Family	2					
Cries				2	1	
Does Not Do as Much for Self as Able			2		2	
Swears						1
Is Dirty						1
Has Inferiority Complex			1			

feel better about caring for "Mom." Admittedly, most of
the aides and other staff at The Nursing Home came from
the same white, working-class backgrounds as the residents;
in fact, the demographic profile of the nurse's aides is
similar to the demographic profile of the residents, tele-
scoped back 60 years. In nursing homes where residents
and staff come from different socioeconomic or racial
backgrounds, those differences may hinder the development of mutual affection.

Extremely unpopular residents may find their tenure
at a nursing home short. This nursing home discharged

415 residents from 1978 to 1984. Half of those residents died, either in the nursing home or in the hospital. Ninety-, nine residents, however, transferred to another nursing home, and a review of their histories suggests that 25 transferred because staff desired the transfer. Nursing homes cannot easily discharge a resident whom staff dislike, but if that resident enters a hospital, the nursing home can refuse to readmit him/her. Indeed, nursing homes often have no vacant bed even for a popular patient returning from the hospital. With an unpopular patient, the nursing home can just as legitimately lack a vacant bed. And, if the bed is actually available, a nursing home may go to a lengthy waiting list, may claim inadequate staffing for the patient's needs, or may simply say no. Some patients gain poor reputations among hospital and nursing home social workers. At The Nursing Home disliked residents often had a brief tenure (4 months median); presumably, staff quickly assessed the prospects for a harmonious relationship.

The Staff

Each state has a nursing home ombudsman, established under the Older Americans Act of 1976. The ombudsman investigates complaints, referring them to diverse regulatory authorities, like the health department. Typical complaints focus on medications, accidental falls, and insufficient physical activity. Families are the usual complainants, although occasionally a physician will contact the ombudsman. In the state where The Nursing Home is located, the nursing home ombudsman received 214 formal complaints in fiscal year 1984. The Nursing Home was not cited.

This clean record on complaints, however, does not signify a staff better trained than those at other nursing homes. Indeed, the importance of training itself deserves some iconoclastic scrutiny. Because nursing homes are funded and evaluated as quasi-hospitals, the credentialling and training standards of hospitals are supposed to apply to them also. But nursing homes are less adequately staffed than hospitals because nursing homes employ a preponderance of aides. In nursing homes, Licensed Practical Nurses and Registered Nurses are in positions of authority, and many nursing homes employ no bachelor's degree or master's degree nurses. Most homes rely largely on unlicensed aides for daily patient care. Although nursing home aides are not especially trained, they are still competent to perform the specific "bed and body routines" essential to patient care. (Indeed, the daughters and daughters-in-law in the community who act as caregivers to their elderly parents rarely have specialized training.) Obviously, some nursing home residents require elaborate nursing techniques, but many do not.

The aides at The Nursing Home perform their duties well, but not necessarily because they know their duties better than aides at other nursing homes. Nor because they are more educated or smarter or more compassionate. They do, however, know their patients. Staff turnover in this nursing home is low. Aides may leave for a time (to get married or have a baby), but will often return, if only part-time. Many tales about inept staff reflect, not nursing inexperience, but inexperience with the specific patients. A nurse new to patients is more likely to administer medications inappropriately, to react unnecessarily to patient movements, to overlook physical changes, to have "accidents" happen when she is helping to toilet or transfer patients. Patient transfers, for instance, happen hundreds of times daily in every nursing home. The worker familiar with Mrs. Smith is comfortable supporting her as she moves from bed to chair. From experience the worker will know how much weight Mrs. Smith can support; and Mrs. Smith for her part will feel comfortable leaning on the aide. With a different aide—not one less familiar with transfers, but one less familiar with Mrs. Smith—an accident is more likely. Similarly, the aide who knows that Mrs. Jones grows dizzy after her children leave will not so quickly panic at a dizzy spell. Staff at The Nursing Home are not extraordinarly credentialled, but they are familiar with their patients; and a satisfied, stable staff familiar with patients may be more critical to patient care than a barrage of inhouse training sessions. Indeed, licensed nurses from a "pool" may be less effective in dealing with patients whom they do not know than would unlicensed aides in regular attendance.

The enthusiastic morale of the staff at The Nursing Home is obvious. In an administration-sponsored survey of staff complaints, many workers requested higher wages and more fringe benefits, but few complained about under-staffing, unclear lines of authority, inattentive administration, or poor work conditions. The home does not hire from agency personnel pools. The home does use part-time staff; but many of these part-timers have worked there previously. Aides studying for a LPN degree may work while attending school. So even the part-time faces are familiar to residents.

In responding to the question about their feelings toward the transfer of specific residents, many staff qualified their responses by stating that they would not want the resident to go to an inferior nursing home. Staff believe The Nursing Home offers wonderful care; indeed, staff who have worked elsewhere praise this facility.

The reasons for the enthusiastic morale are less obvious. To a casual visitor, the nursing home does not look physically superior to any other home. It is clean and orderly, yet unimaginatively sterile. Staff earn the low wages and modest fringe benefits that are the norm for the industry. The home does not reimburse tuition for staff who are studying for degrees. In a proprietary industry where anti-trust regulations prohibit gathering wage information for comparison, a strict benefits comparison is difficult. Ironically, some nursing homes troubled with high staff turnover pay wages above the norm.[12]

One key lies in the director of nurses, who has worked at this facility since it opened in the seventies. According to this state's nursing home ombudsman, the director of nurses sets the tone of a facility. A good director of nurses will understand both residents and staff, will support staff, will be available for help and questions, and will make expectations clear. Unless directions for documenting accidents, questioning medication orders, and referring ill residents to physicians are unambiguous and clear, new staff will often feel stymied. Their confusion will aggravate their frustration when they encounter what they construe as a crisis or a need for a decision. A detached director may foster the sense that standards are not only ambiguous, but unimportant; that the facility is not truly interested in patient care. This nursing home has a committed, sufficiently autocratic director who ensures competent staff performance as well as a fairly satisfied staff. The relationship of staff satisfaction to patient care is cyclic: a satisfied staff will have low turnover, which will lead to greater familiarity of staff with residents, which should lead to more positive staff affect toward residents, which in turn should bolster staff satisfaction.

The Nursing Home is situated in a pleasant working-class neighborhood, accessible by public transportation and convenient to major thoroughfares. Many staff workers live within a ten-minute drive. The home provides a large staff parking lot; and although the home offers no security system for night patrol of the parking lot, the neighbor-

hood is relatively safe. Evening or night staff do not fear
for their safety or their vehicles when they come to work.
Nursing homes in rural areas may find it harder to lure
staff, and homes in urban areas that staff perceive as
dangerous may find it similarly difficult to lure staff.

Toward a New Portrait of Nursing Home Staff

Stereotypes of nursing home personnel linger in part because they corroborate our established notions of nursing
homes. Goffman would have recognized The Sadist or
The Automaton as plausible staff for a total institution.
And when we look at nursing homes through the lenses
of an institutional paradigm, we look for such staff.

The reality, however, is different. In The Nursing
Home the majority of the staff were fond of the majority
of the residents. However alien "staff affect" may be in an
archetypical institution, in this very ordinary nursing home
the staff showed "positive affect" toward residents. Many
residents were generally liked. These residents tended to
be ones who had retained their "historical pasts," where
staff could see them as people, not simply as residents of
West 2 or East 1. And the key to retaining a historical past
lay partially in the secure community niches these residents
had left, their frequent family visitors, and their strong
self-images derived from interesting occupations. These
were people who would not die emotionally alone in the
nursing home. Admittedly, a few residents were disliked,
but their number was small, and interviews with staff
suggested that these residents had, simply, frustrated staff's
desire to feel useful.

The fact that staff desire to feel useful deserves emphasis. Although aides have limited career options, they
do have choices—admittedly, choices among other low-

wage occupations, but choices nonetheless. Their friends and relatives work in factories, mills, retail stores, and restaurants. Aides choose to work in nursing homes; and, as the director of nurses suggested, they generally like helping patients. Anecdotes that describe aides taking residents home for Thanksgiving or to the movies testify to caring, empathetic women.

The charges of an abusive staff, a misanthropic staff, a staff devoid of emotional affect, and an inept staff have been approached sociologically here; and the evidence from The Nursing Home suggests that those stereotypes are not accurate. The aides at this nursing home have minimum education, earn low salaries, and probably have not studied gerontology. They stand in marked contrast to the credentialled sociologists, psychiatrists, bureaucrats, and gerontologists who evaluate nursing home personnel and policies; yet, in this nursing home at least, if the evaluators look, they will see caregivers who give both competent and affectionate care.

Chapter 6

The Myth of Family Abandonment

The images of nursing home abandonment are haunting. In an American retelling of King Lear, the abandoned person sits distraught, waiting for visitors who never come, knitting scarves for grandchildren who rarely write, displaying tattered religious and birthday and New Year's cards from holidays long past. Almost invariably the abandoned resident is a widow who has built a loving family home for a generation of children, who in turn have raised their own families. The truism that "A mother can care for six children, yet six children cannot care for one mother" is a fitting epitaph for the resident deposited in a heartless institution, separated from the family she has nurtured. The woman is invariably sweet, kind, patient, and willing to forgive her errant children if only they would remember her on Mother's Day.

The abandoners present an equally haunting image. Envisioning the frail widow awaiting only a short visit from grandchildren, we conjure up heartless children who will not interrupt their hedonistic pleasures for even an afternoon with Mom. The Biblical commandment exhorts us to "honor thy father and mother: that thy days may be long upon the land which the Lord thy God giveth thee." Children who abandon their parents in nursing homes have violated that commandment. We see those violators as hateful and selfish, and we hope only that they suffer the same fate of abandonment that they have inflicted upon their parents.

The image of familial abandonment is not only haunting, but accepted as legitimate. *The Gin Game's*[1] leading characters, a widow and a divorced man, talk of visitors who never come. The woman's son lives nearby, but does not visit, while the man has lost contact with his children. In fact, no family member visits any resident in *The Gin Game*. Exposes of nursing home scandals reinforce the popular notion that families have simply abandoned their parents. If nursing homes are as filthy, as substandard, as abusive as legislative and newspaper investigations have suggested, then one of three explanations is plausible. Either family visitors are myopic; or they see the abhorrent conditions and do not care; or, finally, they do not visit. The first explanation is ridiculous; the second suggests emotional abandonment; while the third—no visits—reinforces our intuitive fears of physical abandonment.

Our images of abandoned residents, however, may reflect the institutional lenses through which we gaze both at nursing homes and at families. We conjure up pathetic women cruelly overlooked on Mother's Day as heartless children set their family tables with one less setting. This image may be unfair both to nursing home residents and to their families.

A Search for Abandoned Residents

Statistical evidence on the frequency of nursing home visitors is mixed. Although some researchers have found that a majority of nursing home residents regularly receive visitors,[2] other studies[3] have found a sizeable proportion of residents with few or no visitors.

Residents with few or no visitors, however, have not necessarily been abandoned by heartless families. Both hospital and nursing home social workers recognize that general abandonment is a pervasive myth,[4] difficult to scotch.

Even participant observation studies of nursing home life do not support such a myth. In *Limbo* Carobeth Laird[5] laments her isolation, yet concedes that she was estranged from her daughter and grandchildren long before she entered a nursing home. In *A Home Is Not A Home* Janet Tulloch[6] describes the frustration of a middle-aged disabled yet lucid woman living amidst far older, more confused women; yet Tulloch does not dwell on abandonment. Similarly, Jaber Gubrium's[7] description of the social world of a nursing home does not feature distraught residents waiting in vain for mean-spirited children. When nursing home administrator Clifford Bennet[8] described his few days as a nursing home patient, he again did not describe a warehouse of abandoned people.

As for family involvement, the literature suggests that some family relationships may even improve when relatives live in nursing homes.[9] Freed from the stress of constant caregiving, families may be able to offer their relatives "expressive" support, while nursing homes provide the constant "instrumental services.[10] Indeed, some nursing home staff believe some families visit too fre-

quently, in effect discouraging the resident from participating in group activities.[11] Family guilt, not callous
indifference, may be the dominant emotion as families
struggle to reconcile themselves to their own sense that
they have "failed" Mom.[12] Even families who visit regularly, telephone daily, and relay all concerns immediately
to the nursing home administration may feel that they
have "abandoned" Mom although the evidence suggests
the contrary.

The Nursing Home data on visiting patterns permit
a statistical test of familial abandonment. For each of the
130 residents who had lived at The Nursing Home at least
five months, the director of social service, in consultation
with staff nurses when necessary, compiled a record of the
frequency of visits from several different categories of visitors: parents, spouses, children, sibling(s), and extended
family. The five-month minimum benchmark was chosen
so that data would reflect established patterns of family
contact. Residents newly admitted to a nursing home may
have a flood of visitors during the first few weeks, before
the family settles into a pattern. Visits were coded Frequent
(at least once a week); Regular (more than once a month
yet less than once a week); Occasional (less than once a
month yet occasionally), or Rarely/Never. The frequency
of visits was coded numerically. The frequency of visits
from each category of potential visitors was added to form
an Index of Visiting for each resident. Since the Index of
Visiting included different categories of visitors, as well as
the frequency with which any one relative visited, a resident
with several regular visitors would score higher than the
resident with only one frequent visitor. This index became
the dependent variable in a regression equation designed
to isolate variables important in predicting visits.

The independent variables included demographic characteristics of the resident: age, sex, occupation; family characteristics: existence of living relatives (specifically, the existence of a sibling, spouse, or child, constructed as dichotomous dummy variables); tenure within The Nursing Home (all residents who were coded had lived a minimum of five months in the home, so family visiting patterns should have established themselves); prior residence (another nursing home or the community); and patient lucidity (residents were rated as rarely lucid, sometimes lucid, always lucid).

The results suggest that the visited resident, not the abandoned one, may be the norm, at least in this nursing home. Table 6.1 highlights the frequency of visitors.

Table 6.1.   Residents' Frequency of Visitors. (N = 130; Sample A)

Frequent	31%
Regular	56%
Occasional	7%
Never/Rarely	6%

The results also suggest that families are, if not loving, at least dutifully attentive. Table 6.2 outlines the results of multiple regression analysis, with the index of visitors as the dependent variable. The multiple regression equation yielded three major explanatory variables: a living spouse, a living sibling, living children. The betas of living spouse (.36), living sibling (.39), and living children (.35) are strong; and, more importantly, the R^2 of the equation is 45%. In other words, 45% of the variation in visiting patterns was explained largely by the existence of living rela-

Table 6.2.   Regression Analysis, Considering Visits as the Dependent Variable and Resident Characteristics as the Independent Variables. (N = 130; Sample A)

Resident Characteristics	Beta
Living Sibling	.39*
Living Spouse	.36*
Living Children	.35*
Tenure at The Nursing Home	-.15
Admitted from Community	.12
Relatives on Staff	.12
Lucidity	.11
Age	.09
Relatives as Patients	.08
Female	.01
Prior Occupation/Profession	.00

$$R^2 = .45$$

level of significance
    * p .001

tives. At first, the common sense of such a finding mocks the sophisticated statistical technique of regression analysis. Of course residents with relatives are the residents who have the most visitors: the opposite finding would be bizarre. And a statistical confirmation of that wisdom seems unnecessary. Yet, if families have abandoned their mothers and fathers in nursing homes, visiting patterns should not depend so heavily upon families. If familial abandonment exists, in short, the R^2 would be smaller. Clearly the existence of family members would remain the key predictors of family visiting; but the R^2, or the proportion of the variation in visits to be explained by those variables, would be smaller. In a regression equation the error term is the proportion of the variation not explained by the statistical model. In an equation with a high error term, family abandoment would be a feasible explanation.

In this model of visiting, some of the nonsignificant variables merit discussion. Although sociological research generally dwells on significant relationships, Kadushin's proposed *Journal of Nonsignificant Findings* would let researchers air findings whose nonsignificance challenged popularly-accepted notions of social action. In the spirit of such a journal, this model found several variables unimportant in predicting visits; and their lack of importance suggests that popular notions of family relationships may need rethinking.

First, although older patients may outlive their friends and find that their siblings, spouses, even children are unable to visit regularly, this data did not show age *per se* to be a significant deterrent to visitors. In only 2 of these 130 cases were patient families too ill or also institutionalized and thus unable to visit ever; and these patients were not the oldest. As expected, age showed a high negative correlation with the presence of a living spouse (-.29) and a living sibling (-.27); but the direct impact on visits was not strong (-.11). (See Table 6.3 for correlation matrix.)

Second, as expected, women were more likely to survive their husbands and males were more likely to have a surviving spouse. As with age, however, the relationship of gender to visitors lay in the fact that men were more likely to have living wives, not that men would necessarily have more visitors.

Third, prior occupation did not predict patterns of visiting. Although residents with skilled or professional occupations may have had more interesting or less arduous lives than their factory-employed contemporaries, oc-

Table 6.3.   Correlation Matrix of Visits and Selected Independent Variables. (Sample A)

	Age	Sex	Prior Occup.	Tenure	Spouse Alive	Child Alive	Sibling Alive	Lucidity	Visits
Age	—	.02	-.19	.04	-.29	.05	-.27	-.01	-.11
Female		—	-.08	.09	-.37	.10	.07	-.17	-.16
Prior Occupation			—	-.02	.08	-.19	.10	-.16	-.02
Tenure				—	-.11	.03	-.14	.07	-.23
Spouse alive					—	.23	-.02	-.02	.45
Child alive						-	-.32	.04	.30
Sibling alive							—	-.08	.27
Lucidity								—	-.09
Visits									—

cupation did not affect the post-retirement relationships that would be important in predicting visits.

Fourth, patient lucidity did not show a high correlation with visits. Families did not eschew confused or senile patients. Several patients did not recognize their visitors. One man with Alzheimer's disease quacked like a duck and ignored his anguished wife and children on their frequent visits; nevertheless, neither this family nor most of the other families had abandoned their confused relatives.

Nor did family ties diminish with time. Although prior research[13] had suggested that visiting decreased with length of institutional residence, neither tenure in The Nursing Home nor an immediate past residence in a different nursing home showed a strong correlation with level of visits. Over forty percent of residents included in this sample had come to The Nursing Home from a different nursing home, and the median tenure at The Nursing Home was 29 months from the initial admission. (Many patients left for short stays in the hospital, but their tenure was dated from their first admission.) Presumably, families with a relative in a nursing home developed a new kind of homeostasis, incorporating an additional ritual in their lifestyles: the weekly visit.

Toward a Nonparametric Model of Family Involvement

Data from this nursing home cast a statistical barb at the prevalent notion of family abandonment. Nevertheless, the opposite corollary, that families remain deeply committed to their relatives who live in nursing homes, is not valid either. Clearly the involvement of families with institutionalized relatives varies. Some residents have fewer visitors than other residents, or their visitors come less frequently, and the number of family members will not totally explain the difference. Mrs. J.'s husband eats lunch with her every day, staying conscientiously from 11 to 1, helping to feed her, reading her the newspaper, and leaving only when she takes an afternoon nap. On weekends residents' children bring their children to visit. Mrs. X's husband comes twice weekly; her children, occasionally.

Models of family involvement, however, do not lend themselves so easily to statistical computation. We can count the numbers of visitors and the frequency of their visits, but the model that attempts to highlight processes important in predicting involvement would appear to be dealing with nonquantifiable variables. Even though researchers cannot easily measure those variables, however, the variables merit consideration; and a tentative theoretic model of involvement can be posited.

One consideration is the transportation status of "family." Eva W.'s 64-year-old daughter lives a 60-minute bus ride away. In a car, the distance from the daughter's home and the nursing home is 25 minutes; but since the daughter has no car and no convenient access to one, she must take a bus to see her mother. Every few months she makes the trek, even though she herself is not well. The daughter has not abandoned the mother, though; and in frequent phone calls the two keep in touch. If the daughter had a car, if the daughter had a friend with a car, or if the daughter could enlist Senior Shuttle transportation, she would probably be more involved in her mother's care; but, since she cannot change her transportation mode, she remains an occasional visitor. If this nursing home were not accessible by bus, she would be a rare visitor.

Similarly, geographic distance influences family involvement. The Nursing Home is in a working class community where most of the children and grandchildren of the residents continue to live. Elderly people who retire to sunny retirement communities may not expect their children to visit regularly. Hopefully, the retirees will construct pleasurable lives among their contemporaries. Those displanted retirees who enter nursing homes, however, may want visitors, only to find that their children cannot regularly visit. Conversely, children who have moved far from their childhood home may simply be unable to visit often.

Perhaps we need a barometer of affection which will calibrate anger, distrust, disappointment, loyalty, love, sorrow, and so forth. The gerontologists, sociologists, and psychologists who analyze the families of the elderly do not uniformly love their own parents, spouses, or children. And their families do not uniformly love them. Not surprisingly, then, the affections of nursing home residents and their families reflect as wide a gamut of response. The assumption is that a son or daughter neglects to visit an institutionalized parent because the child is cold, heartless, ungrateful, mean, etc. And, of course, the waiting parent is kind, loving, understanding, and patient. The reality is more complex. Some children have not loved their parents; they visit conscientiously out of a sense of dutiful obligation, not affection. And some parents have not loved their children. Familial abuse is not limited to contemporary families. Indeed, one Tennessee physician[14] who surveyed nursing home residents who had returned to their families found that some of them returned to "suboptimal" environments where they were subject to abuse. The emotional bonds of residents and their families were set long before "the nursing home decision," and nursing home residence does not transform residents into martyrs or family members into ogres. Laura G., for instance, has one monthly visitor: a son who lives an hour away. Occasionally his wife and children accompany him; but usually he comes alone, chats for thirty minutes, and leaves. The relationship is cool and distant—a genteel form of abandonment at first glance; yet the relationship has been cordially detached for at least 20-years. Laura and her husband were close to each other. They travelled throughout the country, settling for a time in different spots; and when they grew too frail to care for each other, they entered The Nursing Home together. When her husband died, she lost her anchor to reality. She probably enjoys her son's visits, but the estrangement of decades has made him a distant figure whom she rarely mentions. Joe W. has no visitors, even though his social work chart shows a spouse and children as living relatives. The social work chart also details Joe's years of alcoholism and cycle of admission-discharges to state detoxification programs. Abandonment *has* occurred—though whether he abandoned the family or they abandoned him is arguable. The abandonment, however, occurred long before Joe entered The Nursing Home.

The physical health of relatives belongs in a model of family involvement. Some never-married residents have devoted siblings who are themselves either in nursing homes or unable to visit. Often nieces and nephews will take on a routine of weekly visits to aunts and uncles; but if those same nieces and nephews are caring for their own aged parents, they may be hard-pressed to meet the needs of both parents and extended family. In The Nursing Home several residents sought admission because the relatives caring for them grew too ill to do so. Relatives too ill to give care may be too ill to visit.

The mental lucidity of the nursing home resident also merits attention. In The Nursing Home a 20-year-old girl lies comatose from an infection. For three years her parents have come daily. They talk to her, move her, sit by her side. Her siblings and schoolfriends used to come regularly, but over time they have come less often. Staff marvel at the devotion of the parents, but staff also understand the parents' need to be with their child, even though she gives no sign of recognition or consciousness. A few rooms away a middle-aged woman lies comatose. Her husband, who used to visit frequently, now comes occasionally. He has found a woman friend, presumably one with whom he will attempt to construct a shared life. Staff understand his needs, too. When a nursing home resident is unable to recognize family visitors, those visitors may well not abandon the resident. They may remain involved, yet their intensity of involvement reflects their own needs, not primarily the perceived needs of the resident.

"Competing family interests" belong in the model of family involvement. Families faced with a sick child, unemployment, eviction, delinquency, bankruptcy, divorce, and so on, may rank visiting a relative who at least is safely ensconced in a nursing home, regularly fed, and presumably given adequate medical care a low priority.

The variables posited in a theoretic model of family involvement include: family's travel capability, geographic distance, health, mental status of residents, affection, and competing interests. "Family" itself, however, needs clarification. We expect "family" to remain involved with institutionalized relatives, yet we need to define family ties. The Biblical commandment exhorts children to honor their fathers and mothers. Children's relationships to step-parents can be problematic, however, especially if the child has not lived primarily with the step-parent, has known the step-parent only briefly, or has become a "step-child" in his or her 40's when an older mother remarried. Nor does the Fifth Commandment specify the obligations of extended family—nephews, nieces, cousins, grandchildren, brothers-in-law—to older people. Often nieces and nephews are devoted caregivers to beloved aunts and un-cles, but no societal prescriptions insist that nieces and nephews be responsible for aunts and uncles. As for in-laws, cousins, grandchildren—they may be "family," but the moral obligation of this "family" to be involved remains unclear.

The End of the Search

One hallmark of an institution, as defined by Goffman, is a barrier, either physical or psychological, between inmates and "others." Usually the inmate lives in a world only rarely invaded by others; and the separation of the inmate from the larger society marks a key feature of institutionalization. Architecturally, The Nursing Home does not encourage the integration of "others" into its routine. It has few pleas-ant spots where residents can visit with relatives. Social activities do not concentrate on activities that include families. Indeed, during the time of this research, The Nursing Home had not yet instituted a family support group.

Even in so architecturally unenticing a setting, how-ever, "others" became part of nursing home life. At this nursing home, people with living families are likely to have visitors. The residents who wait for visitors who never come generally have no close living relatives. They may have in-laws, nieces and nephews, and various cousins; but their pre-nursing home relationship with their "extended fam-ily" was never strong enough to compel those relatives to begin a relationship with them once they enter a nursing home. The logistics of travel, the emotional bonds between residents and their families, the health of potential visitors, the consciousness of residents—all may plausibly influence the level of visits; yet, in general, people do not abandon their spouses, their parents, or their siblings.

At this nursing home the search for an abandoned resident ends with a new image: a woman waiting for visitors who conscientiously visit—perhaps not so often as she would like—and who do not abandon her. Indeed, a steady stream of visitors constitutes a key part of a nursing home's ambiance.

A more profitable search for abandonment would focus not on families, but on family physicians, who may well "abandon" their patients once they enter nursing homes. In *Unloving Care*, Bruce Vladeck[15] subtitles his section on physician involvement in nursing homes, "The Missing Physician." Some physicians will no longer treat patients who enter nursing homes,[16] while other physicians visit their institutionalized patients infrequently.[17] Nurses recognize the pen-holding physicians who drop in simply to sign the appropriate payment forms, as well as the hand-waving physicians who poke their heads into patient rooms, wave hello, and then leave. To discourage physicians from ostensibly "examining" a great many patients on one "gang" visit to a nursing home, Medicaid reimbursement regulations limit the number of patients a physician can claim to see on any one nursing home visit. Unlike England, where geriatricians make regular nursing home rounds,[18] the United States has comparatively few geriatricians. American primary care physicians, eager to promote health and rehabilitation, may prefer younger patients to elderly patients, particularly those in nursing homes. In this quasi-medical facility, the visits of physicians do not constitute a key part of the ambiance.

Chapter 7

In Search of
Iatrogenesis

The Greek words "iatro" (physician) and "gennan" (to produce) combine to create "iatrogenic," which has come to mean an additional problem or complication resulting from treatment by a physician or surgeon. Here we will use the word to describe what many people feel is the harmful impact of nursing homes on residents. In nursing homes the minds and bodies of most residents will deteriorate—a deterioration that is a natural function of the aging process. Iatrogenic nursing homes hasten that failure; and people grow sicker, more confused, and less able to function because of nursing home residence.

The professional literature on nursing homes supports the notion of iatrogenesis. Indeed, an archetypal institution by definition is iatrogenic. Residents who experience a "loss of self," "diminished personal autonomy," and "separation from significant others" are expected to grow confused, less competent to function as autonomous adults, more acclimated to the passive role of patient. In nursing homes some residents enter with diminished control, especially if relatives or physicians have made "the nursing home decision" for the resident. Many residents, however, participate in both the decision to enter a nursing home and the choice of home.[1] For these residents the loss of autonomy begins after admission—a loss likely to presage diminished competence. The fact that people who stay more than six months in a nursing home—"long-stayers"—almost never return to the community[2] lends further credence to the theoretical justification for the assumption that the nursing home experience is a harmful one. In fact, one study[3] found that "better" homes discharge more residents—a finding that suggests low discharge rates may be at least partially due to iatrogenic nursing homes.

It has been charged that staff contribute to the iatrogenesis. Trained to perform instrumental tasks on, for, or with residents, staff may regard their charges as "objects of bed and body care." Staff intent on bed and body routines may neglect to offer psychosocial support. One experiment that measured resident functioning when specific nurses engaged in general conversation not necessary for care found that resident functioning improved[4]—a study based on the frightening assumption that casual conversation is unusual. Another study found housekeepers more important sources of emotional support than nursing staff.[5] If aloof staff depersonalize residents, then overzealous staff eager to push wheelchairs, button clothes, and comb hair may "induce dependence" in residents, whose skills will decline in proportion to staff attention. Overly maternal staff who treat residents like children may encourage infantile, incompetent self-images and behavior. Some staff may abuse patients.

The social atmosphere of the nursing home itself may be iatrogenic. Nursing homes' census of confused, depressed, and deranged residents may understandably depress the other residents; indeed, the competent resident may be at a disadvantage.[6] Similarly, the reality of impending death[7] may dominate the nursing home ambiance as residents note the empty beds, the covered stretchers, and the awkward silences from staff. Elderly people in the community also live with the fact that friends and relatives die; but, presumably, the community offers other major events to offset that of loss. In the nursing home every new resident is a potential short-stayer. Short-stayers who return to the community soon after admission remind the other residents that they themselves may not return, while short-stayers who die soon after admission reinforce a pervasive recognition of death as the inevitable, and major, nursing home event.

Residents may even suffer "clinical" iatrogenesis.[8] Residents not forced to walk may become bedridden. Bedridden residents may develop bedsores. Poor hygiene in a congregate setting may contribute to the spread of viral and bacterial infections. Residents served unpalatable, unattractive, non-nutritious food may simply not eat. Untrained staff may administer medications inappropriately or neglect correct procedures for medical crises. One Colorado study that assessed nursing home staff competence to deal with insulin reactions found serious ignorance.[9] Research has similarly documented the persistent phenomenon of inappropriately medicated residents.[10]

Thus, the literature on the effects of institutionalization suggests an inevitable iatrogenesis. Induced dependence, loss of autonomy, clinical mistakes, the status of inmate, poor hygiene—all paint a bleak picture of the nursing home. The search for iatrogenesis within a nursing home promises to be simple because many researchers have portrayed nursing homes as geriatric black holes where people enter, never to return.

A Statistical Tale

Discharge statistics tell a tantalizing tale. The percentages, betas, error terms and correlations present a twentieth century iconography that tells a story; and, like medieval iconography, the numbers evoke a complex story that merits some scholarly probing. Admittedly, researchers can and do manipulate statistics to substantiate their own paradigmatic assumptions about social interaction. With this caution in mind, the statistical findings represent social science icons; and these icons, deciphered, suggest a complex story of discharge and, concurrently, of the extent of iatrogenesis.

Discharge data were gathered on the 415 residents discharged from The Nursing Home from 1978 to 1984. Three discharges are possible. A resident will either:

- Die, either in The Nursing Home or after hospitalization
- Transfer to another nursing home directly from The Nursing Home or after an intermediary hospitalization, or
- Return to the community, directly from The Nursing Home or after hospitalization

The discharge data yield findings that, separately, tell a grim story of decline and death; yet, taken as a whole, suggest that the nursing home may not be so iatrogenic as we may believe.

Finding #1: Most residents admitted to The Nursing Home do not return to the community. The following numbers testify to the reality that Mom has slightly more than one chance in four of returning to the community. She may also transfer to another facility—in fact, 99 of the residents who were studied did so. In their random sample of nursing home patients' careers, Lewis et al.[11] found that only 9% successfully returned home. Of 415 residents discharged in six years of The Nursing Home's operation, three-quarters did not return to the community.

Died	*Transferred*	*Returned to Community*
206	99	110

Many residents of The Nursing Home, however, did not enter the home directly from the community, but had already lived in an institution, as Finding #2 shows.

Finding #2: Almost one-quarter of the residents came from another nursing home, not the community; they are nursing home veterans. Table 7.1 breaks discharge down by preadmission residence. As Table 7.1 shows, almost none of the nursing home veterans returned to the community.

The popular image of an individual just admitted to a nursing home is of a person newly wrenched from community and family. The existence of a sizeable number of nursing home veterans does not mesh with that image.

The popular image also suggests a person leaving a familial home, perhaps one s/he shared with children or a spouse. Again, the reality may not mesh with that image, as Finding #3 suggests.

Table 7.1. Discharge by Preadmission Residence.
(N = 405, Sample C)*

| Pre-admission Residence | Community Discharge to: | | | | | Discharge to Other Institution | Died | Total N |
	Own Home Alone	Own Home With Relatives	Relative's Home	Child's Home				
Own Home	25.7% (57)	9.5% (21)	.9% (2)	3.2% (7)		19.8% (44)	40.8% (91)	100% (222)
Child's Home	1.8% (1)	--	--	23.2% (13)		19.6% (11)	55.4% (31)	100% (56)
Other Nursing Home	1.5% (2)	1.5% (2)	--	2.3% (3)		31.8% (42)	61.4% (78)	100% (127)

*Some cases were missing because records did not indicate patients' preadmission residence.

Finding #3: Most people who returned to the community lived alone. The breakdown of discharge status shows both a surprisingly high proportion of single-occupant households and a surprisingly low proportion of elderly people living with children or relatives, as Table 7.2 shows. Of the 110 people who returned to the community, 60 returned to live alone. The loners, moreover, were not significantly younger than those who returned to live with relatives.

Although some people followed a nomadic path to The Nursing Home (from their own home to an elderly housing complex to a child's home), only 24 of the 110 residents discharged to the community returned to a child's home.

Table 7.2.   Discharge Status of Residents Returning to the Community. (N = 110, Sample C)

Discharge Status	Proportion	Number	Median Age
Own Home Alone	54.5%	60	75
Own Home with Relatives	20.9%	23	76
Child's Home	21.8%	24	79
Relative's Home	2.7%	3	75

Finally, the most important finding is not immediately obvious, but requires content analysis of patient charts.

Finding #4: Most patients who are expected to return to the community do return, while "permanent" residents are never expected to leave. In other words, a patient's initial intake prognosis is central to his/her actual discharge. A nursing home has three discharge tracks, determined at admission and reviewed periodically along with treatment plans. For the discharge prognosis, the physician considers the question, "Can this patient return to the community?" Advised by the admitting physician, the nursing home social worker labels the new resident's prognosis as: "A discharge plan is in progress," "A discharge is uncertain at this time," or "A discharge plan is not in progress." Most states, mandating discharge plans for Medicaid recipients, regularly review the appropriateness of those plans. On the "discharge plan in progress" track are the residents who are expected to go home: this is considered a temporary placement. Usually temporary residents have entered the nursing home for intensive physical therapy or a short convalescence. Some residents have an uncertain discharge prognosis. Their discharge plan is conditional: they may be discharged *if* they recover sufficiently, *if* community agencies will cooperate, *if* the family can find suitable housing. Still other residents, with "no plan in progress," are "permanent" placements.

The discharge prognosis is not based on an elaborate assessment procedure; indeed, critics argue that some residents are incorrectly classified as "permanent."[12] The admitting physician, however, often knows both the patient and the family well; and though the physician may not follow an elaborate multiphasic physical and mental assessment protocol or enlist the help of social workers in recruiting community-based support, the physician's familiarity with the patient and family may be just as important as more scientific assessment criteria in answering the question, "Can this patient be expected to leave the nursing home?"

Table 7.3 highlights the importance of the admission prognosis in predicting the final discharge of 415 residents.

As the numbers show, few of the people—less than 10%—admitted as "permanent" residents returned to the

Table 7.3.   Admission Prognosis Versus Final Discharge Status. (N = 415; Sample C)*

Final Discharge Status	Admission Prognosis		
	Permanent Placement N = 297	Uncertain N = 39	Temporary Placement N = 79
Died	63.5% (188)	38.4% (15)	6.3% (5)
Transferred	28.4% (84)	18.0% (7)	10.1% (8)
Returned to:			
Own Home Alone	2.7% (8)	35.9% (14)	45.6% (36)
Own Home with Relatives	2.4% (7)	2.6% (1)	19.0% (15)
Child's Home	2.7% (8)	5.1% (2)	17.7% (14)
Relative's Home	.7% (2)	--	1.3% (1)

*Discharge was coded according to final status, regardless of hospitalization. People who died or transferred may have been initially admitted to a hospital.

community, while the vast majority—over 80%—of "temporary" residents returned to their community homes.

Discharge was analyzed in a series of related multiple regression equations that point even more emphatically to the importance of the initial prognosis in predicting discharge status. In the first equation, discharge to the community was considered a dependent dummy variable: residents returned to the community or did not. (While, theoretically, nursing home residents who are transferred might at some later date return to the community, realistically they are unlikely to do so. Consequently, transfers and deaths were coded together.) Independent variables included the resident's admission prognosis (coded as negative, uncertain, or positive), gender, pre-admission residence (the community or another nursing home), living relatives, and, most importantly, tenure within this nursing home. In an iatrogenic institution tenure should show a direct effect upon discharge: the longer you stay, the less likely you are to leave. In the second equation, tenure was the dependent variable. In the third equation, the discharge plan was itself considered a dependent variable. All three equations yielded a model of discharge for 1) all people discharged from The Nursing Home (Table 7.4) and 2) all people admitted directly from the community and discharged from The Nursing Home (Table 7.5).

For both samples of residents, the most important variable in predicting discharge is the admission prognosis,

Table 7.4.   Regression Equations for All Residents Discharged from The Nursing Home, 1978–1984. (N = 415, Sample C)

	Dependent Variables		
	Community Discharge	Tenure	Favorable Prognosis
Independent Variables	beta	beta	beta
Family Ties			
Living Spouse	-.04	.01	.04
Living Child(ren)	-.03	-.04	.09
Living Sibling(s)	.04	-.06	.06
Age	-.05	.10	-.11
Sex	.01	.12	.10
Admitted from Community	.09	-.26*	.32*
Favorable Prognosis	.63*	-.16*	--
Tenure in The Nursing Home	-.05	--	--
R^2	.49	.15	.13

significance level
*p .001

with betas of .63 (Table 7.4—sample of all residents) and
.64 (Table 7.5—sample of community residents). Similarly,
a favorable admission prognosis was the key to tenure (-.16)
and (-.20), in that residents with favorable prognoses
tended to have shorter nursing home stays, although the
models predicting tenure were far weaker.

Nonfindings

To offer more material for Kadushin's proposed *Journal of
Nonsignificant Findings,* two nonsignificant independent variables merit attention. First, the presence of family showed
no strong impact either on discharge to the community

**Table 7.5.   Regression Equations for Residents Admitted
from Community and Discharged from The Nursing Home,
1978–1984. (N = 279, Sample C)**

| | Dependent Variables | | |
| | Community Discharge | Tenure | Favorable Prognosis |
Independent Variables	beta	beta	beta
Family Ties			
Living Spouse	-.06	.07	.03
Living Child(ren)	-.05	-.06	.10
Living Sibling(s)	.04	-.13	.07
Age	-.02	.08	-.12
Sex	-.02	.10	.14
Lived Alone	-.04	-.13	-.15
Favorable Prognosis	.64*	-.20*	--
Tenure in The Nursing Home	-.11	--	--
R^2	.47	.09	.08

significance level
*p .001

or on the admission prognosis. We know that supportive families are the major difference between elderly people who live in institutions and those who live in the community. Instinctively, we feel that the presence of family should influence nursing home discharge. We think that people with family supports should be more likely to go home than people without such supports. The evidence does not support that belief. The presence of living family members showed no strong statistical impact on either discharge status or discharge plan.

Finally, the last nonfinding challenges the notion of iatrogenesis: tenure showed no direct relationship to discharge. In an iatrogenic institution, where people grow feebler, more impaired, and more confused as a result of their nursing home experience, tenure should show a strong relationship with discharge status. In the models of community discharge, however, tenure in The Nursing Home showed no significant effect (Table 7.4—the total sample, beta = -.05; Table 7.5—the community sample, beta = -.11). Admission prognosis was the key to discharge; tenure was not. If this nursing home were truly iatrogenic, tenure would have shown a direct positive relationship with discharge; the longer a resident stays, the less likely s/he is to go home; and initial prognosis would not have been the strong predictor it was.

The data on nursing home tenure is complex and seemingly contradictory. At first glance, tenure seems critical because the residents who returned to the community had far shorter stays than the residents who transferred to another nursing home or died in this one. (See Table 7.6 for breakdown of median and mean tenure by discharge status.) Multiple regression analysis, however, allows the researcher to compare the impact, not only of tenure on discharge, but of other potentially important variables.

Table 7.6.   Discharge Status by Tenure in The Nursing Home (N = 415; Sample C)

Discharged to:	Months Tenure	
	Mean	Median
Own Home Alone	4.0	1.4
Own Home with Relatives	3.2	1.9
Child's Home	3.4	1.5
Relative's Home	6.2	2.0
Other Nursing Home	10.7	5.2
Died	14.2	6.6

That comparative analysis suggests that the admission prognosis, not tenure, is the key predictor of community discharge.

The End of a Statistical Search for Iatrogenesis

The statistical findings do not indicate that the residents of The Nursing Home are being harmed by their institutional experience. Instead, the numbers suggest two distinct groups of residents: one group enters as "temporary" residents. The admitting physician, the family, even the resident him/herself expect the nursing home stay to be a short one, and the stay generally is. Often these residents have functioned sufficiently well in the community to live alone; and, even after a nursing home stay, they will return to their own homes alone. Admittedly, they may need community supports; but with those supports they are generally able to manage alone, at least for a while. Later, if they grow ill, they may enter a nursing home as "permanent" placements; but at this stage in their lives the nursing home is a temporary domicile.

The other group enters the nursing home as "permanent." Neither the family physician nor the family expects the resident to return to the community. Their admitting physician calls their placement "permanent," and it generally is. Some of these residents will live for years in this nursing home: the tenure of one permanent resident at The Nursing Home was over five years.

Perhaps "permanent" residents deteriorate partially as a function of nursing home residence; but to determine this social scientists would need to:

• Calibrate the deterioration that would have occurred "naturally" outside of a nursing home; i.e., deterioration considered a normal progression of the individual's aging. People do not always die gracefully or suddenly. Many die slowly, with a concomitant loss of functional ability. Still others suffer from increasingly debilitating diseases, where drugs and therapeutic regimens might retard the debilitation, but will not arrest it. Alzheimer's disease, cancer, multiple sclerosis, Parkinson's disease—all follow a different progression in each individual; yet, except for rare cases of stasis or remission, all follow a progressively worsening course.

• Measure the extent to which institutional features— loss of autonomy, loss of privacy, clinical mistakes, and so on—contribute to the otherwise "natural" decline, i.e., exogenous versus endogenous deterioration. Some policymakers would like to evaluate nursing home performance by feeding the characteristics of the new resident (age and diagnosis, for example) into a computer which, comparing that resident against the statistics for other residents with similar characteristics, would predict that resident's probable life-span, or, more concretely, that person's nursing home tenure. Nursing homes that kept people functioning longer would be deemed praiseworthy and rewarded, while nursing homes where people died before their computer-predicted time would be deemed less praiseworthy—a computer's approach to defeating iatrogenesis.

Unfortunately, we may not yet understand enough about how and why we age to predict our lifespans. Even physicians familiar with their patients might be loath to predict how long a patient will live, and the computerized wisdom of the electronic seer may be no less flawed. Although policy-makers, particularly those eager to gear a financial reimbursement system toward encouraging "better" nursing homes, may construct complex formulas to measure "performance," and, with performance, "iatrogenesis," the formulas will not overcome our inherent ignorance about the timing of death.

Derailed Residents: A Test of Iatrogenesis

Discharge statistics from this nursing home permit one admittedly modest test of iatrogenesis. Although statistics will not reveal the extent to which permanent residents suffer as a result of their nursing home experience, the data on temporary residents permit such a test. In an iatrogenic institution, "temporary" residents would be unlikely to return to the community. Admitted with discharge plans "in progress," these residents would never leave, but would be "derailed." In an iatrogenic nursing home we should be able to trace their derailment directly to their nursing home experience.

Of 79 residents labelled "temporary" upon admission to The Nursing Home, only 13 (16%) did not return to the community. The case histories of these derailed residents offer reasons for their derailment.

Theoretically, "iatrogenesis" would seem the most feasible explanation. Indeed, the literature paints the nursing home as so iatrogenic a place that we probably would expect that more than 16% of "temporary" patients would be derailed.

Other explanations, however, are feasible. First, the physician's answer to the question, "Can this patient return home?" depends partly upon the individual's functional ability, partly upon the requisites of that person's "home." When "home" is a solitary third-floor apartment, the person must be more mobile, more alert, more independent, than when "home" is a bedroom in a child's ranch-style house. Similarly, the "family" will influence the discharge decision. A resident may more easily return to a healthy spouse than to an invalided one. Not surprisingly, discharge "home" to rural areas, which often lack social service supports, is more difficult than to urban ones.[13] During the resident's nursing home stay, his or her "home" may change, mandating a change in the initial discharge prognosis. A family may move or relinquish a parent's apartment. A spouse may die or be hospitalized. If the resident's "home" changes, the resident may be trapped in the nursing home. The entrapment, though, does not result from physicial deterioration or the general effects of prolonged institutionalization, but from the fact that the patient's "home"—one crucial nexus of the discharge plan—has changed.

Caregivers may renege. A potential caregiver must be both able and willing to care for a patient; and willingness does necessarily correlate with the relative's functioning: hospital social workers marvel at the range of families "unable to meet patient needs," as well as at the range of patient disabilities that families find supportable. Some families will care for an incontinent, confused, bedridden patient, while other families demand continence, lucidity, and mobility from the patient. Once a relative has lived in a nursing home, the caregiver may choose to withdraw from that role. In fact, an erstwhile caregiver may relish the reprieve from constant caregiving.

Finally, many residents participate in the decision to enter a nursing home. Weighing life in the community against life in a nursing home, they choose the latter. Notwithstanding the grim popular image of nursing homes, a person may rationally choose to live in one. It offers regular if unimaginative meals, safety from muggers and burglars, companionship, and help with daily activities. Residents who had lived alone may prefer the nursing home even if they could function sufficiently independently within the community. Similarly, residents who planned to return home may change their minds. They may come to value the omnipresent staff, the social ambiance, the safety, even the recognition that they are no longer burdening family caregivers. As Crystal has noted, many elderly people prefer not to depend upon family.[14] Life in the nursing home frees the resident from his/her own guilt. Also, residents subject to abuse and/or neglect at home may find the nursing home a welcome haven.

In sum, patients may be "derailed" because of:

• *Change in Patient Status*
1. A change in physical status, noted by a new or revised medical diagnosis, e.g., a stroke occurring while in the nursing home, the discovery of a tumor, a heart attack. Admittedly, physical status will depend in part upon nursing care, and in specific cases the distinction between clinical iatrogenesis and physical deterioration independent of the effects of the nursing home may blur.

2. A change in overall functioning not directly linked to a specific medical incident. When nursing notes describe the patient as "weak," "apathetic," "no appetite," this is considered a loss of ability to function. Again, the demarcation between a distinct physical change and overall deterioration may be spurious, especially since one may precipitate the other. A patient may fail, not because of institutional iatrogenesis, but because of an undetected change in his or her medical condition. Indeed, a precise delineation between exogenous changes in physical functioning and changes induced by prolonged institutionalization may not be possible. This research, however, seeks to separate changes in family status from changes in patient status.

• *Change in Family Status*
1. Death of caregiver (spouse, sibling, child, extended family).
2. Inability of caregiver (spouse, sibling, child, extended family) to fill role.

• *Patient Chooses to Remain in Nursing Home.*

Critical Events in the Histories of the Derailed

Each derailed resident's chart traced the nursing home history of that resident, from the initial sanguine discharge prognosis to his/her eventual re-classification from "temporary" to "permanent." Table 7.7 summarizes the results.

Two patients chose to remain in the nursing home. One never-married 88-year-old man had previously lived alone in a third-floor apartment. A niece lived on the first floor. After six months, the admitting physician said that the patient could go home. Even though the apartment

**Table 7.7.   Reason for Change in Discharge Status.
(N = 13; Sample C)**

	Number of Residents
Change in Patient Status	
Physical Status	2
Overall Functioning	5
Change in Family Status	
Death of Caregiver	0
Inability of Caregiver to Fill Role	4
(2 caregiver children, 1 caregiver sibling, 1 caregiver extended family)	
Patient Chooses to Remain, Given Option to Leave	2

was still being paid for, the patient decided he did not want to return. He enjoyed the activity and security of the nursing home. An 82-year-old widower, who also had lived alone, had children who maintained his apartment. At the end of two months he chose not to return home, but to transfer to another nursing home, where he had once been a patient.

Four residents' caregivers reneged. One of these residents, a 65-year-old widower, had lived with his sister. His discharge plan specified that he would return to his sister's apartment, but after two months his sister said that she was too ill to care for him. Also, the sister had moved into a one-bedroom apartment which, she explained, was too small for two people. Eventually, after 28 months at The Nursing Home, the patient transferred to a home for veterans. The second person was an 85-year-old widow who had lived in an apartment upstairs from her son was supposed to return to live with that son. Eight months after admission, the patient reportedly called her daughter-in-law to ask to live with her. The daughter-in-law, who had cared for her mother-in-law after two previous nursing home stays, refused. Two months later the patient was admitted to the hospital. She returned to a different nursing home. The third resident was a widow, 81 years old, who was supposed to return to her daughter's home. Five months after admission, the social work case notes reported that neither the son-in-law nor the daughter wanted her to live with them. Three months later the woman died. Finally, the nursing home expected the fourth resident, a 72-year-old never-married woman who had lived alone, to return to her own apartment, where community agencies, assisted and supervised by extended family, would ensure a successful discharge. Since the patient was on a "discharge track," staff encouraged her to walk, bathe, and dress so that she could return home as quickly as possible. After seven days at The Nursing Home, the family complained that staff made the patient do too much. On the family's insistence, the patient transferred to another nursing home. She did not return to the community.

Two residents quickly declined after admission, but the nursing home does not seem culpable. Edith B., an 82-year-old widow with no living children and one sibling, had lived alone. She was admitted with a diagnosis of "bronchial pneumonia and generalized weakness." Five months previously she had been hospitalized for anemia, yet was discharged home alone. This time, the hospital discharged her to The Nursing Home for convalescence. After two months, she was hospitalized and died. Sally M., a 71-year-old widow living alone, but with children nearby, was admitted with an optimistic assessment. Surprisingly, her functional ability declined. Three months after admission, when a tumor was diagnosed, her placement changed to "permanent." One year later she died. Admittedly, both women deteriorated after placement, but their histories do not truly indicate that The Nursing Home was at fault.

Five other residents' functional ability deteriorated, yet their histories also exonerate The Nursing Home. Indeed, one resident improved during his tenure. Adam B., a 62-year-old married laborer admitted from his own home, had suffered a stroke. Staff were supposed to work with him until he could enter a nearby rehabilitation unit. From rehabilitation, he would go home. After eight months in The Nursing Home, he had improved sufficiently to enter the rehabilitation unit, where he did not progress sufficiently to return to the community. After the rehabilitation unit he entered another nursing home.

In retrospect, the favorable prognoses of four of the derailed residents seem unduly sanguine. One 92-year-old widow, living alone, was expected to return to her solitary apartment. Two weeks earlier, she had been hospitalized, yet discharged to her home. After a subsequent hospitalization for electrolyte imbalance and a urinary tract infection, she entered The Nursing Home for convalescence. She stayed two months, was hospitalized, discharged to another nursing home, then tranferred back to The Nursing Home. Six days after readmission she died. A 28-year-old never-married woman, diagnosed as schizophrenic, had a more Panglossian prognosis. After "deinstitutionalization," she lived in a group home, where she became violent and injured herself. She was hospitalized in a psychiatric facility, then discharged to The Nursing Home for convalescence. The social worker expected to discharge her back to the group home because she felt that, regardless of the woman's questionable ability to function in a group home, a geriatric long-term care facility was inappropriate.

Twenty-two days after admission the patient reportedly could not control her "voices." One day later she was rehospitalized, then later transferred to the state mental institution. Another resident, 76 years old, had transferred to The Nursing Home to join his wife. His diagnoses included diabetes, cancer of the colon, leg edema, alcohol abuse, and cirrhosis of the liver. The couple had no children. The man's discharge plan called for him and his wife to live together in their own apartment, assisted by community agencies. After 48 days in The Nursing Home, staff complained that he was abusive. He struck his wife twice. He was discharged to the hospital and from there to the state mental institution. An 81-year-old widow who had lived alone was expected to return home. Staff, though, reported that she did not seem to want to help herself. Since this placement was "temporary," staff recognized her need to practice tasks, yet she did not cooperate, in spite of her professed desire to go home. After five months, both patient and family acknowledged this placement as "permanent." Four months after the change in discharge plan, she went to the hospital for three days. Upon readmission, staff noted she was "relieved to be back in her old room." Her functioning continued to decline. Three months after hospitalization, she would only feed herself, even though staff still felt she could do more. Three months later she died. Clearly, she deteriorated within the nursing home; but nursing notes suggest that staff were trying to slow that deterioration.

Derailing in the Opposite Direction

In addition to the 13 residents who were "derailed" from temporary to permanent status, the records of The Nursing Home show 25 residents derailed in the opposite direction—from permanent to temporary status. While the data already presented here suggest that nursing homes are not necessarily iatrogenic, the data do not suggest the opposite: that nursing home residence per se helps improve residents' functional ability, physical status, and mental lucidity. Although social workers and nurses may cite residents who improved with regular meals, companionship, and clean, orderly surroundings, the case histories of these 25 residents of The Nursing Home do not suggest rejuvenation. An individual entering a nursing home has confronted the inexorable equation of survival needs (admittedly a "need" that varies from individual to individual) against community resources. The histories of these 25 residents testify, not to a change in functional ability or physical status, but simply to a change in the community resources side of the equation—these residents' families had regrouped so that "Mom" could return home. If one caregiver had earlier reneged, another now came forward. If a house was too big and cumbersome for an elderly couple, during their nursing home tenure the family managed to secure a unit in an elderly housing complex. If a disabled individual needed supervision, a housing unit that specialized in apartments for the disabled became available.

Just as the individual's desires entered into the change in discharge status of the other derailed residents, so too the person's own desires explain the change in status of some of these initially "permanent" residents. Individuals who had entered a nursing home because living alone in the community was "too difficult" might simply change their minds. The histories testify to such residents' tenacity in arranging a return to the community. They often telephoned family members, arranged for community services, and contacted neighbors. Sam E. displayed that tenacity. Sam had been admitted from the hospital, which was reluctant to discharge him "home" to his third-floor room in a boarding house; and, since he had no family, the admitting physician labelled the placement permanent. After six months in The Nursing Home, however, Sam wanted to leave. He telephoned his former landlady, arranged for a friend—also elderly—to help him move, and waited until the landlady had a vacant first-floor room, which she agreed to hold for him. When a room was vacant, he returned "home."

Unfortunately, the histories do not document what happens to these "derailees" unless they seek re-admission—as many do. Sylvia X. had lived with a succession of her children, all of whom vacillated between guilt at leaving their mother in a nursing home and distraught agony at having her live with them. Her history consisted of hospitalizations, followed by nursing home convalescences, followed by return to a child's house. On admission to The Nursing Home, the physician labelled the placement "permanent" because the exhausted family believed they lacked the patience, the time, and the energy to be caregivers to a very irascible, independent, 82-year-old woman. After a few months in The Nursing Home, she convinced the family to remember their guilt, not their exhaustion; and they consented to take her "home." Within six hours the family telephoned The Nursing Home, pleading with the director to take their mother back.

Some families may recognize that readmission to a nursing home is inevitable, yet choose to take "Mom" home nonetheless. One 70-year-old woman with Alzheimer's disease had lived at The Nursing Home for a year when her 45-year-old daughter chose to take her home. The daughter did not think The Nursing Home was mistreating or neglecting or abusing her mother; she simply wanted to care for her mother, even though she had to relinquish her paying job as a nurse to become an unpaid nurse for a woman who ostensibly did not recognize her, who needed constant supervision, and whose eventual deterioration would, the daughter conceded, propel her back to a nursing home once again. Some staff questioned the daughter's rationality; other staff marveled at her filial dedication.

A Noniatrogenic Institution

The notion of a noniatrogenic institution seems as much an oxymoron as "nursing home," yet neither the statistical evidence nor residents' histories support the notion of nursing home iatrogenesis. Nursing homes are institutions with routines that allow little patient autonomy. Residents are primarily "patients." Staff perform instrumental tasks on, for, or with residents. Some staff may unwittingly promote dependence or infantilize residents. With ill people clustered in one building, residents are susceptible to bacterial and viral infections. Except for those people who use the nursing home only for a short convalescence, all residents deteriorate. In this nursing home, three-quarters of the residents did not return to the community.

The admitting physicians, however, did not expect most of these people to return home. Of the more than 400 residents discharged in six years of this nursing home's life, 79 entered with favorable prognoses. Only 13 were derailed—and case histories do not suggest that The Nursing Home was to blame.   If one assumes that nursing homes may be iatrogenic for those with uncertain or negative prognoses, one could theorize that the other 66 residents may have escaped comparatively unscathed because they stayed only a short while, or because staff may treat "temporary" residents differently from "permanent" ones, or because they themselves saw their role of patient as short-term and hence avoided the "loss of self" endemic to institutional life. These 66 residents, however, did not noticeably suffer from their nursing home stay—a finding that contradicts the presumption of iatrogenesis.

Chapter 8

Conclusion

This book began as a research journey through an ordinary nursing home, but a journey that asked onlookers to discard their customary lenses. We are accustomed to seeing nursing homes through lenses that reflect a dominant paradigm of institutions, a Manichaean dichotomy of family versus nursing home, and, finally, our aversion to the thoughts of death that nursing homes evoke.

The new lenses reflected a "family" paradigm. Instead of probing the extent to which nursing homes strip residents of autonomy, induce dependence, increase social isolation, and deplete self-esteem, this research investigated the extent to which residents form bonds with those around them, retain their prior identities, and retain ties with family. It also investigated the extent to which staff developed affection for residents. In short, the research searched for familial aspects of nursing homes. Any investigation into social reality reflects a specific mind-set. Presumably, researchers with "noninstitutional" mind-sets might find positive aspects of the nursing home experience that researchers with "institutional" mind-sets had overlooked. The nursing home, its residents, its staff, its administrative policies remain the same, but different lenses yield a different image.

This research was conducted in a 160-bed nursing home that was not designed by an architect interested in promoting interaction among the elderly. The two-bed rooms allow little privacy, and the few communal rooms do not invite intimate visits with family. Nor does The Nursing Home have an affiliation with a gerontological center or a university medical school. The home's social activities consist of the usual routine of bingo, meals, prayer and sessions with the hairdresser. In the background, televisions whir. Staff are largely unlicensed aides. No experimenters are trying, with plants, birds, or pets, to promote independence. The Nursing Home looks, sounds, and smells like many of its counterparts.

Yet even in this unexceptional nursing home, a change of lenses yielded a portrait that is less harsh, less frightening than the massive amount of negative literature would suggest.

In this nursing home most residents who could communicate found a friend. Loners tended to be people unable to communicate lucidly. The friendships did not mirror the class and ethnic cleavages so important outside the nursing home; but age-contemporaries befriended each other. If Mom can communicate with others, she may find that the nursing home represents, not exile from the community, but a place where she can make new friends.

Although some people became "cases," forfeiting their past identities, the data suggest that residents with frequent visitors and interesting past occupations are less likely to suffer that fate. Mom will not necessarily shed her identity to become the "case in Room 106."

Staff at The Nursing Home were neither sadistic nor unfeeling. The majority of staff were fond of the majority of residents; and staff who knew something about a resident's past were more likely to develop feelings of affection for him or her. Although some residents were unpopular, they were few in number; and the anecdotes about unpopular residents are more than balanced by the anecdotes of staff who informally adopt residents, taking them on outings or to meet their families. Mom may well find caring, conscientious people among the staff. Mom will not die emotionally alone.

Families continued to visit. The residents with no visitors tended to be residents with no immediate families. Families may not have visited as frequently as residents might have wanted: the logistics of travel, illness, competing demands on time, and the strength of the affection all doubtless influenced the intensity of families' commitment; nevertheless, families remained a regular nursing home presence. If Mom had strong bonds with her children before she entered the nursing home, those children will not abandon her.

Finally, the evidence did not support the contention of nursing home-induced deterioration. Residents who were expected to return to the community generally did. Few residents were "derailed" from their initial discharge prognosis; and the social work histories of those few cases exonerate The Nursing Home. If Mom enters a nursing home with a positive prognosis, she will probably leave. The nursing home is not a geriatric black hole where those who enter never return. If they do not return, the reason does not lie in the iatrogenic institution.

In a nursing home, family members are replaced by hired custodians as primary caregivers; yet the evidence from this nursing home suggests that they offer conscientious, compassionate care. Indeed, the more that families recognize staff, not as hired underlings paid to perform "bed and body work," but as genuine caregivers, the more positive the nursing home experience will be for Mom. This research highlighted staff-family interaction as central. Families who visit frequently, who chat with staff about their relative, and who thank staff for their attentiveness are likely to find that staff will look upon Mom as a person with a past, not simply as a case. If Mom is irascible, belligerent, and violent, the family that pointedly commiserates with staff, that shows some compassion toward them, and that occasionally expresses gratitude may help distraught staff better serve an otherwise "difficult" patient. Indeed, staff members often grow fond of Mom; and when she leaves, they will miss her.

A Lament for the Community

Research set within an institutional paradigm has spurred researchers, gerontologists, and policy analysts to mystify "the community" into a social organism that is inherently better than the horrid nursing home. Much as plants will not survive in barren soil, so too people will not survive in a setting as bereft of affection, love, and stimulation as the nursing home. When we see rows of wheelchair-bound people lining the corridors of a nursing home, we blame the nursing home for a lack of stimulating activities, for a routinized schedule, for callous staff who treat residents like warehouse cargo.

Policy-makers have accordingly reified "the community" into the salvation of these wheelchair-bound nursing home denizens. The goal has become, not to make nursing homes more familial, but to strengthen residents' "community homes" so that they might return to them. Community supports—adult day care, Meals on Wheels, homemaker services, visiting nurses, friendly visitors—are to bolster the resources available to the elderly person. Not only will community-based care be inherently better, but it will also be cheaper, or so policy-makers hope. Where such policies are widely accepted, families can be encouraged, prompted, even forced to keep Mom with them.[1]

When we look at the wheelchair-bound nursing home residents lining the corridors, however, we might focus, not on their setting—the nursing home rather than the community—but on the residents themselves. They are ill. Their career, to paraphrase one researcher, is death.[2] The most ebullient staff, the most varied social schedule, the most delightful aesthetic decor may well make these people enjoy their lives more, but changes in setting will not alter the real physical and mental deterioration of the residents themselves. When we focus on the setting and overlook the people, we get a skewed image of the nursing home. Researchers, aghast at inhumane mental institutions, spearheaded campaigns for "deinstitutionalization," even though some mentally ill people truly needed a structured, sheltered environment. So, too, researchers determined to move people out of nursing homes may be overlooking the physical and mental limitations that cause people to enter a nursing home.

"The community" is not an elixir that will in and of itself retard the career of death. Indeed, for many nursing home residents "the community" was "iatrogenic." Some residents who lived alone had difficulty preparing meals, cleaning their homes, going to doctors' appointments, and monitoring their medications. Some residents lived with caregivers who themselves needed care. Residents who depended upon children often stayed home alone during their children's eight-hour workdays. Although ostensibly living with "family," they were emotionally isolated for most of the week. Some residents came to the nursing home after a nomadic trek, beginning with their own home, then to an apartment in an elderly housing complex, then to one child, then to another. If a primary caregiver became ill, married, divorced, moved, or died, Mom would begin the exodus to a new caregiver.

The siren song of "strengthened community resources" reverberates in discussions of long-term care options. Clearly, with sufficient resources, some people might return to their communities; and, once returned, some of those people might thrive. Social workers have anecdotes of such success stories. These success stories, however, may not be the norm; and when we glorify these tales of rejuvenation, we may be offering a distorted image of the larger nursing home population. A walk through The Nursing Home reveals many severely incapacitated people unlikely to thrive in "the community."

Indeed, the nursing home itself is a community; and researchers eager to improve the lives of residents might concentrate, not only on keeping people out of nursing homes, but on developing loving, humane, caregiving communities within them. Nursing homes are already regulated; but those regulations largely apply medical, dietary, and safety standards to a place that purports to offer a home. (And those health and safety regulations, moreover, often set low standards.) Regulations that address social, aesthetic, and emotional standards might help transform these quasi-medical facilities into homes.[3]

A *Lament for Independence*

The last lament is for the loss of independence that plagues nursing home residents, who depend upon others for physical survival. Staff prepare meals, help toilet, push wheelchairs, guide walkers, operate bathtub lifts, give backrubs, button clothes, fill water pitchers. Scales of "activities of daily living" mirror children's mastery of "independence skills," from walking to toileting. Residents present a marked contrast to people who can eat, bathe, dress, and move independently.

Nursing home residents, however, also need friendship, affection, humor, companionship, stimulation; and in that social dependence residents do not differ markedly from the rest of us. Indeed, parents who have served the needs of their "dependent" children often depend upon those children for joy and meaning. We all depend upon one another. In 1624 John Donne meditated that, "No man is an island, entire of itself"—a thought so often cited it seems a truism, yet a truism that people yearning to restore nursing home populations to "independence" may overlook. Perhaps technological fetishism has obscured the human interdependence that John Donne noted, but it cannot obscure the truth of what he said. Nursing home residents, families, staff, gerontologists, sociologists—we are all bound to one another. In helping one another, physically and emotionally, we affirm our common humanity. Our zeal to help the elderly person live "independently" may reflect the darkened lenses through which we gaze.

References and Notes

Chapter One

1. M.B. Norton: Liberty's Daughters: The Revolutionary Experience of American Women, 1750-1800. Boston: Little, Brown & Co., 1980.
2. J. Tey: The Daughter of Time. New York: Macmillan, 1952.
3. T. Kuhn: The Structure of Scientific Revolutions. Chicago: University of Chicago Press, 1970.
4. J.D. Watson: The Double Helix. New York: Atheneum, 1968.
5. E. Goffman: Asylums. Garden City, NY: Anchor, 1961.
6. A. Strauss (ed.): George Herbert Mead on Social Psychology. Chicago: University of Chicago Press, 1964.
7. A sampling of germane research includes:

    N.N. Anderson: Effects of institutionalization on self-esteem. *Journal of Gerontology* 22: 313-317, 1967.

    R. Bennett: The meaning of institutional life. *The Gerontologist* 3: 117–125, 1963.

R. Bennett: Social context—a neglected variable in research on aging. *Aging and Human Development* 1: 971, 1970.

M. Baker: Reasons and cure for dehumanization in nursing homes. *Hospital and Community Psychiatry* 25: 173–174, 1974.

R.M. Coe: Self-conception and institutionalization. In: A.M. Rose and W.A. Peterson (eds.), Older People and Their Social World. Philadelphia: F.A. Davis, 1965.

R.L. Kane and R.A. Kane: Alternatives to institutional care of the elderly: Beyond the dichotomy. *The Gerontologist* 20: 249–259, 1980.

M.A. Lieberman: Institutionalization of the aged: Effects on behavior. *Journal of Gerontology* 24: 330–340, 1969.

J. Wack and J. Rodin: Nursing homes for the aged: The human consequences of legislation-shaped environments. *Journal of Social Issues* 34: 6–21, 1978.

8. F.E. Moss and V.J. Halamandaris: Too Old, Too Sick, Too Bad. Gaithersburg, Maryland: Aspen Systems Corporation, 1977.

9. K. Kesey: One Flew Over the Cuckoo's Nest. New York: Signet, 1975.

10. *Going in Style (film: U.S. Warner)*, Martin Brest, Director, 1979.

11. W.H. Jarrett: Caregiving within kinship systems: Is affection really necessary? *The Gerontologist* 25: 5–10, 1985.

12. J.A. Burgun: Integrated housing for the elderly. *Journal of Public Health Policy* 4: 64–68; 1983.

13. S. Crystal: America's Old Age Crisis. New York: Basic Books, 1982, pp. 45–51. Crystal suggests that living through the Depression with aged parents shaped

some of the attitudes of contemporary elderly people, who do not want to burden their children or forfeit their privacy.

14. M. Smallegan: Decision-making for nursing home admission: A preliminary study. *Journal of Gerontological Nursing* 7: 280–285, 1981.

   F. Beland: The decision of elderly persons to leave their homes. *The Gerontologist* 24: 179–185, 1984.

   P. Townsend: The Last Refuge—A Survey of Residential Institutions and Homes for the Aged in England and Wales. London: Routledge and Kegan Paul, 1962.

   S. Tobin and M. Lieberman: The Last Home of the Aged. San Francisco: Jossey-Bass, 1976. Tobin and Lieberman argue that many elderly people begin to feel the impact of "institutionalization" when they make the nursing home decision, even if they do not enter a nursing home immediately.

15. E. Brody: Patient care as a normative family stress. *The Gerontologist* 25: 19–29, 1985.

   M.H. Cantor: Strain among caregivers: A study of experience in the United States. *The Gerontologist* 23: 597–604, 1983.

16. M.F. Browning and H. Shore: Preparing a visitors' guide for family members—some considerations. *Concern* 1: 20–22, 1975.

17. G. Lienhardt: Divinity and Experience: The Religion of the Dinka. London: Oxford University Press, 1961.

18. P. Aries: The Hour of Our Death. Hammondsworth: Peregrine Books, 1983.

19. Franklin to Benjamin Vaughn, Nov. 2, 1789. In A.H. Smyth (ed.), Writings (10 vols)., New York, 1905-

1907, Vol. 10, pp. 49–50. Cited in D. Fischer: Growing Old in America. The Bland-Lee Lectures Delivered at Clark University. New York: Oxford University Press, 1977, p. 67.

20. B. Isaacs, M. Livingstone, and Y. Neville: Survival of the Unfittest. Boston: Routledge & Kegan Paul, 1972.

21. G.M. Hopkins: "Spring and Fall." In: Poems of Gerard Manley Hopkins, Third ed. New York & London: Oxford University Press, 1948, p. 94.

22. B. Vladeck: Unloving Care: The Nursing Home Tragedy. New York: Basic Books, 1980.

23. M.A. Mendelson: Tender Loving Greed: How the Incredibly Lucrative Nursing Home "Industry" Is Exploiting America's Old People and Defrauding Us All. New York: Alfred A. Knopf, 1974.

24. J. Hendricks, V. Change, B. Hetzl, and E. Kahana: Correlates of expanded and contracted relationships in homes for the aged. Detroit: Wayne State University, Elderly Care Research Center, n.d.

25. N.B. Epstein, D.S. Bishop, and S. Levin: McMaster model of family functioning. *Journal of Marriage and Family Counseling* 4: 19–31, 1978.

D. Olsen, D. Sprenkle, and C. Russell: Circumplex model of marital and family systems: Cohesion and adaptability dimensions, family types, and clinical applications. *Family Process* 18: 3–28, 1979.

D. Kantor and W. Lehr: Inside the Family. San Francisco: Jossey-Bass, 1975.

Chapter Two

1. B.B. Manard, R.E. Woehle, and J. Heilman: Better Homes for the Old (Lexington, Mass.: D.C. Heath: 1977, p. 21.

2. B. Vladeck: Unloving Care: The Nursing Home Tragedy. New York: Basic Books, 1980, p. 151.

3. M. Devitt and B. Checkoway: Participation in nursing home resident councils: Promise and practice: *The Gerontologist* 22:49–53, 1982.

4. B. Vladeck: Unloving Care: The Nursing Home Tragedy. New York: Basic Books, 1980, p. 23.

5. L. Withers-Borth, J. Hashimi, and E. Rathbone-McCuan: Selfhood of elderly women in a nursing home context. Paper presented at Annual Meeting, American Public Health Association, November 1982.

6. E. Sherman and E.S. Newman: The meaning of cherished personal possessions for the elderly. *Journal of Aging and Human Development* 8: 181–192, 1977.

   S.K. Holzapfel: The importance of personal possessions in the lives of the institutionalized elderly. *Journal of Gerontological Nursing* 8: 156–158, 1982.

   P. Millard and C. Smith: Personal belongings: A positive effect? *The Gerontologist* 21: 85–90, 1981.

7. The home employs more people; the figures cited reflect research conducted during the summer of 1982 when all day and evening shift full-time staff who had worked at The Nursing Home at least four months were interviewed.

8. J.N. Henderson: Nursing home housekeepers: Indigenous agents of psychosocial support. *Human Organization* 40:300–305, 1981.

9. B. Vladeck: Unloving Care. New York: Basic Books, 1980, pp. 17–19.

10. B. Isaacs, M. Livingstone, and Y. Neville: Survival of the Unfittest. Boston: Routledge & Kegan Paul, 1972.

11. S. Tobin and M. Lieberman: Last Home of the Aged. San Francisco: Jossey-Bass, 1976.

12. B. Vladeck: Unloving Care. New York: Basic Books, 1980, pp. 147–162.

13. K.G. Engelhardt: Keynote Address, Northeastern Gerontological Society, Fifth Annual Meeting, Boston, Massachusetts, April 25, 1985.
14. G.J. Tulloch: A Home Is Not a Home. New York: Seabury Press, 1975.

Chapter 3

1. T.S. Eliot: "Choruses from 'The Rock,'" Collected Poems 1909-1962. New York: Harcourt Brace Jovanovich, Inc., i, 1963, p. 154.
2. D.L. Coburn: "The Gin Game." New York: Samuel French, Inc., 1978.
3. P. McGinty and B. Stotsky: The patient in the nursing home. *Nursing Forum* 6: 238–261, 1967.
4. T. Parsons: Definitions of health and illness in light of American values. In: E.G. Jaco (ed.), Patients, Physicians and Illness. 2nd ed. New York: Free Press, 1973, pp. 197–227.
5. S. Marks: Multiple roles and role strain: Some notes on human energy, time and commitment. *American Sociological Review* 42: 921–936, 1977.
6. F. Wiltzius, S.R. Gambert, and E.H. Duthie: Importance of resident placement within a skilled nursing facility. *Journal of the American Geriatrics Society* 29: 418–421, 1981.
7. S. Crystal: America's Old Age Crisis. New York: Basic Books, 1982, p. 69.
8. Participant observation studies testify to the existence of friendships among nursing home residents.
    C. Bennett: Nursing Home Life: What It Is and What It Could Be. New York: The Tiresias Press, 1980.

C. Laird: Limbo. Novato, CA: Chandler & Sharp, 1979.

J. Gubrium: Living and Dying at Murray Manor. New York: St. Martin's Press, 1975.

G.J. Tulloch: A Home Is Not a Home. New York: Seabury Press, 1975.

9. J. Hendricks, V. Change, B. Hetzl, and E. Kahana: Correlates of expanded and contracted relationships in homes for the aged. Detroit: Wayne State University Elderly Care Research Center, n.d.

10. M.F. Lowenthal and C. Haven: Interaction and adaptation: Intimacy as a critical variable. *American Sociological Review* 33: 20–30, 1968.

11. T. Bell: Relationship between social involvement and feeling old among residents in homes for the aged. *Journal of Gerontology* 22: 17–22, 1967.

S. Bergman and I.O. Cibulski: Environment, culture, and adaptation in congregate facilities: Perspectives from Israel. *The Gerontologist* 21: 240–246, 1981.

H. Weihl and I. Ashkenazie: Satisfaction of old age home residents with the home. *Gerontologia* 11: 66–75, 1975.

12. D.B. Miller and S. Beer: Patterns of friendship among residents in a nursing home setting. *The Gerontologist* 17: 269–275, 1977.

L. Wells and G. Macdonald: Interpersonal networks and post-relocation adjustment of the institutionalized elderly. *The Gerontologist* 21: 177–183, 1981.

13. R. Kane and R. Kane: Assessing the Elderly: A Practical Guide to Measurement. Lexington, M.A.: Lexington Books, 1981.

14. Although the home has 160 beds, only 145 patients

were sufficiently established in the minds of staff to figure into a diagram of interaction. Also, some patient days are lost due to hospitalizations.

15. I.J. Firestone, C.M. Lichtman, and J.R. Evans: Privacy and solidarity: Effects of nursing home accommodation on environmental perception and sociability preferences. *International Journal of Aging and Human Development* 11: 229–241, 1980.

E.P. Friedman: Spatial proximity and social interaction in a home for the aged. *Journal of Gerontology* 20: 566–570, 1966.

D.C. Jones: Spatial proximity, interpersonal conflict and friendship formation in the intermediate care facility. *The Gerontologist* 15: 150–154, 1975.

M.P. Lawton and B. Simon: The ecology of social relationships in housing for the elderly. *The Gerontologist* 8: 108–115, 1968.

L.E. McClannahan: Therapeutic and prosthetic living environments for nursing home residents. *The Gerontologist* 13: 424–429, 1973.

16. N.L. Chappell: Informal support networks among the elderly. *Research on Aging* 5: 77–99, 1983.

17. R. Kane and R. Kane: Assessing the Elderly: A Practical Guide to Measurement. Lexington, MA.: Lexington Books, 1981, pp. 166–167, 197–198.

18. E. Cumming and W.E. Henry: Growing Old: The Process of Disengagement. New York: Basic Books, 1961.

19. I. Rosow: Social Integration of the Aged. New York: Free Press, 1967.

20. G. Arling: The elderly widow and her family, neighbors, and friends. *Journal of Marriage and the Family* 38: 757–768, 1976.

N.D. Glenn and S. McLanahan: The effects of offspring on the psychological well-being of older adults. *Journal of Marriage and the Family* 43: 409–421, 1981.

G. Lee: Children and the elderly: Interaction and morale. *Research on Aging* 2: 367–391, 1980.

J.A. Mancini: Family relationships and morale among people 65 years of age and older. *American Journal of Orthopsychiatry* 49: 292–300, 1979.

S.R. Sherman: Patterns of contacts for residents of age-segregated and age-integrated housing. *Journal of Gerontology* 30: 103–107, 1985.

21. A. Hochschild: The Unexpected Community. Berkeley, CA.: University of California Press, 1978.

Chapter 4

1. A Strauss (ed.): G. Herbert Mead on Social Psychology. Chicago: University of Chicago Press, 1964.

2. T. Parsons: Definitions of health and illness in light of American values. In: E.G. Jaco (ed.), Patients, Physicians and Illness. 2nd ed. New York: The Free Press, 1973.

3. C. Laird: Limbo. Novato, CA: Chandler & Sharp, 1979.

4. J. Weiss: Nurses, Patients, and Social Systems: The Effects of Skilled Nursing Intervention upon Institutionalized Older Patients. Columbia, MO: University of Missouri Press, 1969.

5. J.N. Henderson: Nursing home housekeepers: Indigenous agents of psychosocial support. *Human Organization* 40:300–305, 1981.

6. C. Kadushin: Response to Antonovsky article. *Sociological Inquiry* 37: 323–332, 1967.

Chapter 5

1. K. Kesey: One Flew Over the Cuckoo's Nest. New York: Signet, 1975.
2. C. Stannard: Old folks and dirty work: The social conditions for patient abuse in a nursing home. *Social Problems* 20: 329–342, 1973.
3. Center for Disease Control: Impact of policy and procedure changes on hospital days among diabetic nursing home residents—Colorado. *Morbidity and Mortality Weekly Report* 33: 621–629, 1984.
4. S.S. Handschu: Profile of the nurses' aide: Explaining her role as psycho-social companion to the nursing home resident. *The Gerontologist* 13: 315–317, 1973.

   M. Baker: Reasons and cure for dehumanization in nursing homes. *Hospital and Community Psychiatry* 25: 173–174, 1974.

   J.S. Kayser-Jones: Old, Alone and Neglected. Berkeley: University of California Press, 1981.

   G. Shuttlesworth, A. Rubin, and M. Duffy: Families versus institutions: Incongruent job expectations in the nursing home. *The Gerontologist* 22: 200–208, 1982.

   J. Gubrium: Living and Dying at Murray Manor. New York: St. Martin's Press, 1975. Gubrium used the phrase "bed and body work" to describe nursing tasks.
5. M.L. Gresham: The infantilization of the elderly: A developing concept. *Nursing Forum* 15: 195–210, 1976.

   R. Bennett: The meaning of institutional life. *The Gerontologist* 3: 117–125, 1963.

6. The literature on induced dependence is substantial. Specific experiments at giving residents control over something (a bird feeder, for instance) demonstrate that residents are more alert when the environment encourages them to behave responsibly. Some examples include:

J. Avorn and E. Langer: Induced disability in nursing home patients: A controlled trial. *Journal of American Geriatrics Society* 30: 397–400, 1982.

M.M. Baltes and E.M. Barton: Behavioral analysis of aging: A review of the operant model and research. *International Journal of Behavioral Development* 2: 297–320, 1979.

M.M. Baltes and M.B. Zerbe: Independence training in nursing home residents. *The Gerontologist* 16: 428–432, 1976.

M. Baltes, S. Honn, E. Barton, M-J. Orzech, and D. Lago: On the social ecology of dependence and independence in elderly nursing home residents: A replication and extension. *Journal of Gerontology* 38: 556–564, 1983.

E. Barton, M. Baltes, and M-J. Orzech: Etiology of dependence in older nursing home residents during morning care: The role of staff behavior. *Journal of Personality and Social Psychology* 38: 423–431, 1980.

G. Banziger and S. Roush: Nursing homes for the birds: A control-relevant intervention with bird feeders. *The Gerontologist* 23: 527–531, 1983.

E.J. Langer and J. Rodin: The effects of choice and enhanced personal responsibility for the aged: A field experiment in an institutional setting. *Journal of Personality and Social Psychology* 34: 191–198, 1976.

P.B. Lester and M.M. Baltes: Functional interdependence of the social environment and the behavior of the institutionalized aged. *Journal of Gerontological Nursing* 4 (2): 23–27, 1978.

M. MacDonald and A.K. Butler: Reversal of helplessness: Producing walking behavior in nursing home wheelchair residents using behavior modification procedures. *Journal of Gerontology* 29: 97–101, 1974.

S.O. Mercer and R.A. Kane: Helplessness and hopelessness in the institutionalized aged: A field experiment. *Health and Social Work* 4: 90–106, 1979.

M.A. Mikulic: Reinforcement of independent and dependent patient behaviors by nursing personnel: An exploratory study. *Nursing Research* 20: 162–165, 1971.

K. Solomon: Social antecedents of learned helplessness in the health care setting. *The Gerontologist* 22: 282–287, 1982.

7. R.L. Kane and R.A. Kane: Long-term care: A field in search of values. In: R.L. Kane and R.A. Kane (eds.), Values and Long-Term Care. Lexington, MA.: Lexington Books, 1982, p. 15.

8. N. Ikegami: Institutionalized and the noninstitutionalized elderly. *Social Science and Medicine* 16: 2001–2008, 1982.

9. G.A. Hotz: Nurses' aides in nursing homes: Why are they satisfied? *Journal of Gerontological Nursing* 8: 265–271, 1982.

R.Y. Pablo: Job satisfaction in a chronic care facility. *Dimensions in Health Services* 53: 36–38, 1976.

H.T. Brown, J. Soloman, and R. Tappen: A symposium on long-term care. *Journal of Gerontological Nursing* 8: 9–15, 1982.

10. W. Watts: Social class, ethnic background and patient care. *Nursing Forum* 6: 155–162, 1967.

11. T. Aries: Issues in the psychiatric care of the elderly. In: A.N. Exton-Smith and J.G. Evans (eds.), Care of the Elderly: Meeting the Challenge of Dependency. New York: Grune & Stratton, 1977, p. 77. "For the nurses incontinence was not the most burdensome nor the most disagreeable disability—it was the morose, uncommunicative patients that they least enjoyed nursing and if a patient was outgoing and cheerful—what was often called "a character"—almost no disability was too burdensome to the staff . . ."

12. H.M. Waxman, E.A. Carner, and G. Berkenstock: Job turnover and job satisfaction among nursing home aides. *The Gerontologist* 24: 503–509, 1984.

Chapter 6

1. D.L. Coburn: The Gin Game. New York: Samuel French, Inc., 1978.

2. R.A. Spasoff, A.S. Kraus, E.J. Beattie, D.E.W. Holden, J.S. Lawson, M. Rodenburg, and G.M. Woodcock: A longitudinal study of elderly residents of long-stay institutions. 1. Early response to institutional care. 2. The situation one year after admission. *The Gerontologist* 18: 281–292, 1978. This study found that after one year in a nursing home, 94% of residents regularly saw relatives.

National Center for Health Statistics. The National Nursing Home Survey: 1977 Summary for the United States. Vital and Health Statistics. Series 13, No. 43, DHEW (PHS) PU61. 79–1794. Washington: USGPO, 1979. This study found 61% of residents had a visitor at least once a week.

W.F. Hook, J. Sobal, and J.C. Oak: Frequency of visitation in nursing homes: Patterns of contact across the boundaries of total institutions. *The Gerontologist* 22: 424–428, 1982. Surveying visitors on three consecutive Sundays in three nursing homes, the authors found 54% of residents had at least one visitor.

3. D.B. Miller and S. Beer: Patterns of friendship among patients in a nursing home setting. *The Gerontologist* 17: 269–275, 1977. In one nursing home the authors found 26 of the residents had no visitors.

   T.J. Curry and B.W. Ratliff: Effect of nursing home size on resident isolation and life satisfaction. *The Gerontologist* 13: 295–298, 1973. The authors found residents in smaller homes had fewer relatives and fewer visitors than residents in larger homes.

   D.E. Gelfand: Visiting patterns and social adjustment in an old age home. *The Gerontologist* 8: 272–275, 304, 1968. The author found the average resident had two visitors every few weeks.

4. R. Greene: Families and the nursing home social worker. *Social Work in Health Care* 7: 57–67, 1982.

   L. Romney: Extension of family relationships into a home for the aged. *Social Work* 7: 31–34, 1962.

5. C. Laird: Limbo. Novato, CA: Chandler & Sharp, 1979.

6. G.J. Tulloch: A Home is Not a Home. New York: Seabury Press, 1975.

7. J. Gubrium: Living and Dying at Murray Manor. New York: St. Martin's Press, 1975.

8. C. Bennett: Nursing Home Life: What It Is and What It Could Be. New York: The Tiresias Press, 1980.

9. K.F. Smith and V.L. Bengston: Positive consequences

of institutionalization: Solidarity between elderly parents and their middle-aged children. *The Gerontologist* 19: 438–447, 1979.

E. Litvak: Three bases for practice. In: M.R. Dubrof and E. Litvak (eds.), Maintenance of Family Ties of Long-Term Patients: Theory and Guide to Practice. Department of Health and Human Services, Publ. 81–400, Washington, D.C.: USGPO, 1981.

M.B. Miller and A.P. Harris: Social factors and family conflicts in a nursing home population. *Journal of the American Geriatrics Society* 13: 845–851, 1965.

R.J.V. Montgomery: Impact of institutional care policies on family integration. *The Gerontologist* 22: 54–58, 1982.

10. G. Shuttlesworth, A. Rubin, and M. Duffy: Families versus institutions: Incongruent job expectations in the nursing home. *The Gerontologist* 22: 200–208, 1982.

11. M.F. Browning and H. Shore: Preparing a visitors' guide for family members—some considerations. *Concern* 1: 20–22, 1975.

12. S. Cath: The geriatric patient and his family. *The Journal of Geriatric Psychiatry* 5: 25–46, 1972.

13. W.F. Hook, J. Sobal, and J.C. Oak: Frequency of visitation in nursing homes: Patterns of contact across the boundaries of total institutions. *The Gerontologist* 22: 424–428, 1982.

14. J. Powers: Nursing home discharges in clinical practice. *Journal of the Tennessee Medical Association* 76: 777–779, 1983.

15. B. Vladeck: Unloving Care: The Nursing Home Tragedy. New York: Basic Books, 1980, pp. 17–19.

16. J.B. Mitchell: Physician visits to nursing homes. *The Gerontologist* 22: 45–48, 1982.

17. R.N. Ballard: The trouble with nursing homes. *Postgraduate Medicine* 72: 307–308, 311, 1982.

18. J.S. Kayser-Jones: Old, Alone and Neglected. Berkeley: University of California Press, 1981.

Chapter 7

1. M. Smallegan: Decision-making for nursing home admission: A preliminary study. *Journal of Gerontological Nursing* 7: 280–285, 1981.

   F. Beland: The decision of elderly persons to leave their homes. *The Gerontologist* 24: 179–185, 1984.

   S. Tobin and M. Lieberman: The Last Home of the Aged. San Francisco: Jossey-Bass, 1976.

2. R.L. Kane, R. Bell, S. Riegler, A. Wilson, and E. Keeler: Predicting the outcomes of nursing home patients. *The Gerontologist* 23: 200–206, 1983.

   E.B. Keeler, R.L. Kane, and D.H. Solomon: Short and long-term residents of nursing homes. *Medical Care* 19: 363–370, 1981.

   K. Liu and K.G. Manton: The characteristics and utilization pattern of an admission cohort of nursing home patients. II. *The Gerontologist* 24: 70–76, 1984.

   J.F. Van Nostrand: The aged in nursing homes: Baseline data. *Research on Aging* 3: 403–415, 1981.

3. M.W. Linn, L. Gurel, and B.S. Linn: Patient outcome as a measure of quality of nursing home care. *American Journal of Public Health* 67: 337–344, 1977.

4. J. Weiss: Nurses, Patients, and Social Systems: The Effects of Skilled Nursing Intervention Upon Institutionalized Older Patients. Columbia, MO: University of Missouri Press, 1969.

5. J.N. Henderson: Nursing home housekeepers: Indigenous agents of psychosocial support. *Human Organization* 40: 300–305, 1981.

6. J. Posner: Notes on the negative implications of being competent in a home for the aged. *International Journal of Aging and Human Development* 5: 357–364, 1974.

7. V.W. Marshall: Socialization for impending death in a retirement village. *American Journal of Sociology* 80: 1124–1144, 1975. Marshall suggests that the fact of impending death may unite residents.

8. D.G. Campbell: Prevention of infection in extended care facilities. *Nursing Clinics of North America* 15: 857–868, 1980.

   I. Gurevich: Infected decubiti: The problem of patient placement and care. *Topics in Clinical Nursing* 5 (2): 55–63, 1983.

   F.T. Sherman, V. Tucci, L. Libow, and H. Isenberg: Nosocomial urinary-tract infections in a skilled nursing facility. *Journal of the American Geriatrics Society* 28: 456–461.

9. Center for Disease Control: Impact of policy and procedure changes on hospital days among diabetic nursing home residents—Colorado. *Morbidity and Mortality Weekly Report* 33: 621–629, 1984.

10. J.L. Segal, J.F. Thompson, and R.A. Floyd: Drug utilization and prescribing patterns in a skilled nursing facility: The need for a rational approach to therapeutics. *Journal of the American Geriatrics Society* 27: 117–122, 1979.

11. M.A. Lewis, S. Cretin, and R.L. Kane: The natural history of nursing home patients. *The Gerontologist* 25: 382–388, 1985.

12. S. Allison-Cooke: De-institutionalizing nursing home patients: Potential versus impediments. *The Gerontologist* 22: 404–408, 1982.
13. K. Supiano and N. Peacock: Discharge planning for residents of a long-term facility. *Quality Review Bulletin* 7: 17–25, 1981.
14. S. Crystal: America's Old Age Crisis. New York: Basic Books, 1982.

Chapter 8

1. E. Brody: Parent care as a normative family stress. *The Gerontologist* 25: 19–29, 1985. "The call for filial responsibility masks social irresponsibility, disadvantaging the elderly and young as well as the middle generation."
2. E. Gustafson: Dying: The career of the nursing home patient. *Journal of Health and Social Behavior* 13: 226–236, 1972.
3. A. Munley, C.S. Powers, and J.B. Williamson: Humanizing nursing home environments: The relevance of hospice principles. *International Journal of Aging and Human Development* 15: 263–284, 1982.

Although the nursing home in which the research for this book took place did not wish to be named, interested professionals and researchers can contact the author through the publisher for the name.